WHY DID I COME INTO THIS ROOM?

WHY DID I COME INTO THIS ROOM?

A CANDID CONVERSATION ABOUT AGING

JOAN LUNDEN

THORNDIKE PRESS
A part of Gale, a Cengage Company

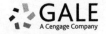

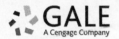

GALE
A Cengage Company

Copyright © 2020 by Joan Lunden.
All photos not otherwise credited are from the author's personal collection.
Thorndike Press, a part of Gale, a Cengage Company.

Thorndike Press® Large Print Nonfiction.
The text of this Large Print edition is unabridged.
Other aspects of the book may vary from the original edition.
Set in 16 pt. Plantin.

LIBRARY OF CONGRESS CIP DATA ON FILE.
CATALOGUING IN PUBLICATION FOR THIS BOOK
IS AVAILABLE FROM THE LIBRARY OF CONGRESS

ISBN-13: 978-1-4328-7858-0 (hardcover alk. paper)

Published in 2021 by arrangement with Forefront Books

Printed in Mexico
Print Number: 01   Print Year: 2020

I dedicate this book to my female readers. This book was written because of you. All of you who spent your mornings with me for the two decades as I hosted *Good Morning America,* my morning friends; I hold you close to my heart. All of you who connect with me day in and day out on my social media platforms sharing your concerns and your own stories have become an extended family of sorts. And to all of you whom I have met as I've crisscrossed this nation speaking at events, thank you for your continued support.

I know it's a giant cliché, but we are truly in this boat together. As women, we experience aging differently than our male counterparts. It is a journey that can leave us feeling frightened, frustrated, and alone at times. I want to shine a light on those dark moments that would then help us all feel more empowered and less alone.

Women fuel my passion to research and learn more about how we can better care for our health and our happiness in order to age more successfully. You have sent me on this mission, to seek the answers to those questions that each of us individually might be embarrassed to talk about.

In addition to seeking answers, I felt compelled to start an open dialogue about aging in this country. As I discuss in this book, aging has changed dramatically, and we need to be better prepared. An open dialogue will help us understand how our female bodies function and the changes that naturally come with the aging process. It can also serve to remind us all that there is a silver lining to aging: reflection, gratitude for a life well lived, time for more relaxation, and new opportunities for many of us. It is up to us to replace the dismal expectations of aging with an anticipation of enjoyment and, yes, even excitement if you plan it that way. That is the mindset that I ask you to hold as you read this book.

Again, women are all in this boat together, and we can learn from one another and take strength from one another. As I wrote this book, I never lost sight of my purpose to empower you, to give you tools, and, yes, to give you a laugh now and then, and to make sure that none of you feel you were on this aging journey alone. You most certainly are not.

Joan

TABLE OF CONTENTS

9

PART TWO: BODY

PART THREE: SOUL

INTRODUCTION:
AGING AIN'T FOR SISSIES!

"The wisdom acquired with the
passage of time is a useless gift
unless you share it."
— ESTHER WILLIAMS

I had a hair-raising experience a while back
that sent shivers up and down my spine. I
was sitting in my office ready for a scheduled
phone interview with *The Hollywood Reporter.* I had done many interviews with
them over the years, especially during my
time at *Good Morning America.* But now, I
was doing special reports for the *Today*
show and this interview was to promote one
of our upcoming series on the Baby Boomer
generation. It was about the importance of
social connections as we age and the power
of having friendships.

As soon as the reporter said hello, I
noticed that he sounded rather young. But
that didn't surprise me as much as the first

question he asked. He began, *"So Ms. Lunden, what will it be like for you returning to morning TV as a senior citizen?"*

I felt like asking if my mother was on the call with us. Instead, I sat stunned. I sat silently for a moment, doing my best to regain my composure.

I'd never been called a *senior citizen* before, nor had I ever thought of myself as one. I didn't want to come across as defensive, but I couldn't help feeling a little shocked by the realization that he saw me that way — aka *old*!

Did it sting? Like a bee.

Talk to me when your facial hair starts growing!

Thankfully, he moved on.

Clearly, I did not.

It happened a few years ago, yet I'm still thinking about it (thankfully, not hourly or daily anymore, only weekly).

It happened a few years ago, yet I'm still thinking about it.

And why is that? I guess because it dawned on me that this young man googled me, saw that I was in my 60s, and then *labeled* me accordingly. It made me think: What else does that automatically make me in his eyes? A *has-been*? Someone who is no longer relevant in today's youth-obsessed

14

world? Or maybe just too old to be a woman on TV?

It felt as though there was a hidden implication that I should be frightened. Or maybe they should build a chairlift on set for me or my own motorized scooter. I wasn't scared; I have faced cancer head on and survived it. I have 7 children. I have interviewed some of the most amazing people in the world. I could handle this age thing. Bring.It.On.

Okay, so maybe I'm a little oversensitive about being called a *senior citizen.* I mean, technically, I do fit the age requirement. Even so, I don't feel like one. Whenever I receive mail marketed to me as a senior, I trash it. It can't hit the receptacle fast enough. Sometimes I'll shove it way down to the bottom of the bin so no one else will see it.

Life Alert offer? Nope. Not mine.

Someone *obviously* made a mistake sending it to me, and if it stays in my possession too long, I fear it might rub off on me.

Oh no. How long do I have before "A Place for Mom" calls to ask if I need "A place for me"?

I must confess that, although I reacted to the reporter's comment this way, the jarring start to our interview really got me thinking

15

about age and ageism.

The word "old" is almost a dirty word in our society. While I definitely feel older, I absolutely don't feel old, and I certainly have no shame about my age. It is, after all, just a number. It might not be the lowest number, but it's definitely not the highest number either.

When it feels like someone is calling you out as a senior, as it clearly did with that young reporter, it can sound as if you have some horrible contagious disease that makes everyone look at you differently — almost with pity. It's an awful feeling. One I regret giving any credence to when it happened. But let's be honest; it happens. I'm human. Could this insecurity I was feeling be fostered by our culture's inherent fear of aging? I'm certain of it.

I found myself wondering, *When exactly did I pivot in other people's minds from being a normal, active, contributing member of society — capable of competing with the rest of the population — to a card-carrying senior citizen?* Why did that have to make me less than? Especially when I know I am still very capable of contributing to the world, especially in some ways more capable than I have been before. Have you ever been confronted with an experience that left you feeling this way?

On the bright side, senior citizens get numerous financial benefits from the government, and they even enjoy discounts from private companies. So, yeah, we get to pay a little less at the box office to see a movie and can take a larger deduction on our taxes. Thank you very much. But at what cost? I worry that this could mean I won't be welcome in line with everyone else who still wants or needs to work, make a difference, be relevant, or even just buy hip clothes and get away with wearing them unjudged.

Our society always seems so focused on youth. Advertisers, fashion designers, even car manufacturers routinely target this market. Because youth is so highly valued, it's almost natural to assume that getting older is something to be *devalued.*

In other parts of the world, seniors are revered for their knowledge and their life experience, whereas our Western culture seems to view humanity the same way we view products: Use while still fresh, then ditch for something newer and fresher. I just don't want to be viewed as having outlived my shelf life. *That stinks,* especially when I know I have so much more to give.

Writing about my life always feels a bit

like laying on a psychiatrist's couch. It forces me to dig deep, to delve into the scary places where my fears and worries reside, and to reflect on the choices I've made so far. I mentally put myself there because I believe that sharing our journeys — including our personal stories, the mistakes we've made, and the lessons we've learned — may help others, or at the very least, amuse them. I've often been guided by the wonderful quote that follows:

> "You don't inspire others by being perfect. You inspire them by how you deal with your imperfections."
> — UNKNOWN

For this reason, I've shared some of my most personal and difficult challenges with viewers and readers over the years. My last big overshare, as you will recall, was in 2014 when I was diagnosed with breast cancer. *People* magazine asked me to appear on their cover bald for that story. *Bareheaded* bald — as in no scarf, no hat, no vanity. As I contemplated writing this book I thought, *If I could muster up the nerve to do that, I think I can share just about anything.*

So here I am, nearly three decades and eight books after the release of my first publication, sharing my innermost thoughts about the very latest issue I'm coping with today . . . *Aging.*

Of course, this means I must be willing to admit in print (and aloud for all of you listening to the audio version of this book) that I am concerned about the aging process and must also confide how I'm faring in that process.

Fortunately, it also means I get to explore and make the distinction between *being older* and *being old,* not just for the benefit of those of us at a certain age, but for readers of every age.

■ ■ ■ ■

PART ONE: MIND

■ ■ ■ ■

"Aging is mind over matter
If you don't mind, it doesn't matter."
— MARK TWAIN

PART ONE
MIND

"Aging is mind over matter.
If you don't mind, it doesn't matter."
— MARK TWAIN

Chapter 1
How Old Would You Be If You Didn't Know How Old You Are?

"Age is something that doesn't matter,
unless you're a cheese."
— Billie Burke, American Actress

What is age, really? Is it as important a description of who we are as most people would have us believe? Or is it just a number on a piece of paper that reflects the moment in time when we were born?

Our Western culture is careful to document everyone's birth date and to use that information to help characterize us throughout our years. But did you know that there are places in the world where the concept of age doesn't even exist? I visited one such place nearly two decades ago, and I must say, it had a profound effect on me that has lasted all these years.

I wanted to take my three eldest daughters, Jamie, Lindsay, and Sarah, somewhere during their high school spring break that was totally different from anywhere else they had ever been. They were teenagers at the time, and I knew they'd be *leaving the nest* soon. My aim was to open their eyes to the many different ways people live and to stir in them an appreciation for those differences. I knew exactly where to take them . . . Morocco.

This mother-daughter adventure began in Casablanca, a bold, bustling city teaming with mosques and colorful bazaars. From there we drove into the Moroccan countryside toward the more ancient cities of Rabat and Fez. It took almost a day of travelling through some of the most extraordinary mountains and gorges to reach a small town called Erfoud, which you might call the last outpost of Moroccan civilization since it literally sits at the edge of the Sahara. There, we got into yet another vehicle — a 4 × 4 — which took off into the legendary dunes of remote Znigui where the shapes of the landscape constantly shift with the winds.

On our first night in the desert, we enjoyed a traditional Moroccan dinner and rested in elaborate tents that were lined with brightly colored tapestries and dotted with tiny crystal beads that twinkled in the moonlight. It was like the interior of a beautiful genie bottle. We were glamping before it was popular!

We awakened before dawn to mount camels for a 30-minute ride out to a sand dune where we would watch the sunrise over the Sahara. The thought of sharing this exquisite moment with my daughters was overwhelmingly joyous. I knew we'd never forget sharing such an experience together.

It was still dark as we emerged from our tents. We could barely make out the silhouettes of the camels, a dozen of them, all laying down in a row waiting for us. In order to protect us from blowing sand our guides wrapped our heads with large colorful scarves so that only our eyes were exposed. For anyone who hasn't ridden a camel before, the process of getting on them is pretty weird. Once you're on board, the camels first raise up their back legs so that you feel like you're going to topple forward right over the camel's head, and then they get their front legs up from under them. It takes a moment to feel stable and secure, but it's really cool once you do.

Our camels began to quietly walk single file through the soft sand with nothing but dunes in front of us until finally the caravan stopped. We dismounted our camels, and the guide pointed to the top of a dune. We started climbing. Once at the top, we sat and waited.

Sunrise in the Sahara. It was an unforgettable experience that, no doubt, we will all remember as long as we live.

It was so worth the wait!

I am really glad we didn't have phones with cameras, Instagram, Facebook, or Twitter back then. It allowed us to live in the moment, and to experience events with our eyes and not through our cameras. Today it would be very hard to do that.

Once back on the road, as desert turned into flatland, our guide spotted a tribe of nomadic Bedouin sheepherders. With the hope of possibly meeting them, he pulled over to the side of the road.

He struck up a conversation and they explained that they move with the changing seasons, picking up their tents and belongings and taking them all with them through the desert and surrounding mountains from one location to the next. When our guide asked if they would mind showing us their home, they were happy to oblige.

Upon entering one of their tents, we were greeted by a warm and welcoming older woman who seemed to be the matriarch of the family — perhaps she was the grandmother. It was hard to determine her age as her skin had been quite weathered by the harsh desert sun and wind. I can still recall her face. She would've made a compelling subject for a sunscreen ad in our country. In her country she was just quite strong and beautiful.

When we spoke with her, we mostly talked about her family and her children. Ultimately, I asked her how old she was.

The woman looked at me as if she didn't know what I was talking about.

I reiterated my question through our translator and the woman explained that they had no clocks, no calendars, and that they lived their lives according to sunrises, sunsets, and the seasons. No one knew their age.

It was an eye-opening moment.

So how old was she?

Did it matter?

Obviously, it didn't.

Was there a lesson to be learned from her response? It certainly made *me* question why age matters so much to us in the Western world.

What that elder Bedouin tribeswoman said in that Moroccan tent that day changed my view of age forever.

When we returned home from our trip, I took stock of the way we measure our lives

— of how we mark the years in annual Hallmark moments — and I started asking, *Why?*

We celebrate every twelve months with a party, and, of course, with another birthday card. And as we get older, those cards joke more and more about sagging body parts, faulty memory, and, of course, about being *over the hill.*

Is that *really* funny?

Oh, and let's not forget the cake with the ever-increasing number of candles to blow out. Is it necessary to include *all* of them? You would think that at some point it becomes a bona fide fire hazard! And how about those people who think it's hysterical to buy the candles that won't extinguish? You blow them out and they light up again and again. Thanks, now I'm a year older *and* about to pass out. Always funny to gaslight an elder who keeps assuming she did, indeed, blow them out.

Don't even get me started on the tradition of following the "Happy Birthday" song with the verse, "Are you one? Are you two? Are you three . . . are you *sixty-seven?*" Yeah, that gets less and less funny as the years pass. Although I will admit, it was cute when the little ones sang it at my father-in-law's recently celebrated 85th birthday.

Well, maybe not to him.

Why is this even acceptable? Your birthday shouldn't be humiliating or embarrassing; after all, we don't give a seven-year-old a card that says, "We are glad you were born, but you're too small and don't know enough to be of any use yet." We don't keep candles off a sixteen-year-old son's birthday cake because he crashed a car and we tell him, *You can't be trusted with fire.* We don't seek to make people feel uncomfortable when they're young, so why would we do it when they're older?

I'm not sure when we started describing our abilities, our strengths, and even our sexual appeal in terms of our age. Or when we started saying things such as, "I look good . . . for my age."

Who needs a qualifier like that?

Certainly, the weathered tribeswoman in Morocco didn't! That brave woman, who would pull down the tent, tie up all of her belongings, and set out into the desert guided only by the sun and the stars whenever the seasons changed, would have no time for such nonsense. That inspiring woman, who had never received a birthday card telling her she was too old to keep her family and her tribe moving, would be appalled. I'm certain she never said, "I gather

29

everything up and move our entire camp like a 20-year-old." She just does what must be done.

I don't know about you but I kind of envied her and her way of living!

If I am being completely candid, I've always hated birthdays. Especially since that trip to Morocco. They just feel unimportant and annoying to me. In fact, I have come to believe that if they are *not* a celebration of everything we are and everything we are still capable of becoming, they are actually *bad* for us. They can affect our psyches, our opinions of ourselves, and worse — they can negatively impact our expectations, our continuing personal growth, and the further development of our abilities.

Of course, none of us is likely to move into a tent in the desert anytime soon, but could we if we didn't know our age? I think we could. Why must we immediately question ourselves? "I'm in my 60s; should I really be galivanting about the Sahara and moving the entire camp? Shouldn't I be moisturizing in this desert climate and taking it easy?" Why can't we try to be a little less preoccupied with our age according to our birth certificate? I believe we can, and that's one of the reasons I've written this book. To get us all rethinking the subject of age and its meaning in our lives.

So how would *you* answer the question: How old would you be if you didn't know your age?

Have you ever thought about it before?

Go ahead and contemplate it now. Ask yourself how old you *feel,* how old you think you *look,* or more simply, how old you are *in your mind.*

What's your number?

If you're like most people, that age is probably younger than the age according to your birth certificate. In fact, for most of us it's a lot younger.

I've done this exercise with many different people and they are often taken aback at first. But they eventually settle into an age that feels right for them. If they are past 50, I find that they almost always pick an age that is at least ten years younger than their actual age.

For those of you who imagine yourself to be older than you are, there may be mitigating factors, such as your current state of health, but I certainly hope that you didn't respond that way because society has convinced you that you are older than you are.

Psychologists say that how we perceive ourselves has a huge influence on how we present ourselves. It impacts how we conduct our lives and what we think we can do. For most of us, it's something we're not even conscious of.

> "The trouble is, when a number — your age — becomes your identity, you've given away your power to choose your future."
> — RICHARD J. LEIDER

Wow. If this is true, then our actual age isn't really as important as the age we picture ourselves to be. The age we feel we are — more than our biological age — can greatly impact our future, the goals we allow ourselves to set, and the strides we have yet to make.

Okay, then age is just a number that can change depending on who's asking.

Today, I pick 45. That's my story and I'm sticking with it!

As we age, we focus on being younger, just as when we were growing up, we longed to be older. I can remember being a little kid dreaming about becoming a teenager. Thirteen seemed like such a magical age; I couldn't wait to get there. And once I hit thirteen, sixteen became the desired age, because then I could drive a car. Older girls just seemed so much cooler than me. Sixteen came and went, and you likely know the next part of this story; twenty-one was the goal so I could vote and drink . . . well, legally. Ironically, the year I turned 21 the legal voting age was lowered to 18 and most states followed by dropping the legal drinking age to 18.

It wasn't until my 20s that I generally loved my age. I enjoyed being a young adult. I was beginning my career in broadcasting, living in my own place, and feeling as if the world was my oyster. I had all the perks of being an adult but was still young enough that older women would call me "youthful" and "fresh-faced." Those years were a time of life filled with so much freedom. There were no children or responsibilities yet and so much possibility and excitement were still awaiting me. At that point in my life, aging was the last thing I was thinking about.

As we progress through the years, people seem to be bothered the most with those passages measured in decades. Turning 30, 40, 50, 60, and so on becomes a significant milestone.

I wasn't bothered at all with turning 30. I was a first-time mom, had an awesome new job as the host of *Good Morning America,* and life was great. How could I possibly be bothered by that? I didn't really mind turning 40, either, since it was a seminal time in my life. I had taken back control of my weight and, in turn, my health and energy level. I had exited a marriage that made me feel as though I had put my life on hold for a long time, and I was now a single working mother who was free to make life decisions on my own. I wanted to have fun and start dating again, which, by the way, was a very eye-opening experience.

When you date after divorce, you suddenly feel just as anxious and awkward as a teenager. You question the outfit you're wearing, the small talk you're making, and whether you should even sit through the entree when you realize at the appetizers that this guy is not for you! That's when I learned to always meet for a coffee first before accepting a dinner invitation.

Even if I didn't enjoy dating all that much, I loved my 40s and the wonderful experiences it brought to my life. But when I was staring down 50, things began to change. That was a much scarier milestone

Did turning 50 signify half-time? Why did that have to make me feel "less than" when I know I'm still very capable of contributing to the world? In some ways, more capable than I have been before. Was I now *over the hill*? Does it all go *downhill* from here? People are living longer in this country than they ever have before. Your 60s is just not over the hill anymore. It's more like the top of the hill. And guess what? We can see clearly from up here. We can reflect back on the journey it took to get here, with all its potholes and challenges, and we can be proud of ourselves. We can look forward to a new us that's yet to arrive. Party supply stores line their shelves with all kinds of paraphernalia suggesting that's the case. Sure, it's funny when you're 20. So why then must we still have one of those awful banners looming over our office cubicle with a bouquet of black roses beneath it and your colleagues are shouting, "Surprise!" Because party supply stores line their shelves with all kinds of nasty rhetoric suggesting that we are over the hill, that our vitality is gone, and that it's all funny.

Most people I know in their 50s today are more active and full of life than some millennials I know. They work out with a vengeance, eat healthily, take care of their bodies, do yoga or meditate to stay calm, and they love adventure. Is this who marketers are looking at when they are producing those *Over the Hill* cards, banners, and birthday mugs? I doubt it.

Maybe 50-year-olds felt over the hill twenty years ago, but it seems to me that things are very different now. Everyone knows 50 is the new 30, 30 is the new 20, and 20 is the new 10. Wait, wasn't that a movie? Say hello to my little friend, Benjamin Button. Seriously, I want to start a picket line in front of party supply stores to make their management take a good look at who we really are. Are you with me?

While I rather enjoyed turning 40, and eventually came to terms with the big 5-0, I didn't completely cherish turning 60. So I asked myself that question: *How old would you be if you didn't know how old you are?* For me, the answer is still 45. That's *my* number . . . apparently that's where I got off the age train.

> "All your life you think 60 is ancient, and all of a sudden, you find you're 60 and you don't really feel that different. I feel stronger and more engaged. This is the best time of my life."
> — GLENN CLOSE

CHAPTER 2
SIX SURE SIGNS I'M AGING

"Why do they say we're over the hill?
I don't even know what that means and
why it's a bad thing. When I go hiking
and I get over the hill, that means I'm
past the hard part and there's a snack
in my future."
— ELLEN DEGENERES

When I first began writing books, I had a wonderful agent, Al Lowman, may he rest in peace. Each time I would turn in a manuscript I remember telling him that I felt as if I had squeezed every last thought out of my head to write it. "Now what?" I'd ask. "Would I have another book to write?" He told me that I would never go wrong if I always wrote about the subjects I wanted to know more about. Today, that leaves me writing about *aging.* I want to understand the process, its effects, and everything else about it so that while it's happening, I can be proactive about my total health — mind, body, and soul.

Although I live my life by the 60-is-the-new-40 rule, I don't kid myself. I know that I am aging. Here are the six sure signs of it:

1. I Still Love Facing a New Day, But I No Longer Bound Out of Bed the Way I Used To.

When I wake up these days and put my feet on the floor, I feel my body unfolding slowly, straightening little by little, until I am fully upright. As I raise my head, press my shoulders back, take that first tenuous step, and become more erect, I find myself chuckling because the whole standing routine reminds me of the chart that used to hang in every American grammar school classroom. It depicts the evolutionary development of man (aka, Homo sapiens). You know the graphic, but in case you're having a *senior moment* — LOL — I'm including it here. The next time you inch your way to the bathroom in the morning, think about this graphic, and tell yourself, "I'm evolving into the age I want to be . . . 45". At least you'll be able to start your day with a laugh. If that doesn't work, say to yourself, "Joan Lunden is having the same thought as me this morning!"

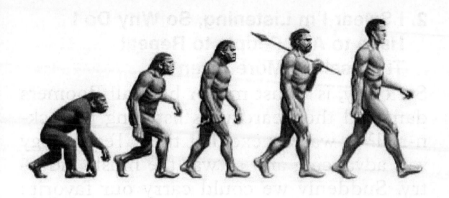

What's really crazy is that once I stopped waking up before sunrise to do early morning TV, I could have kicked back, put my feet up, and taken life easy. Instead I jacked up my work and travel schedules, remarried, and had two sets of twins (twenty months apart!), which kept me rising before dawn for many more years. So much for sleeping in!

As it turns out, I've discovered that as we age, we tend to wake up earlier. Some people say it has to do with our circadian rhythms, but I know it's because we must pee and we can't hold it until morning! But we'll talk more about weak pelvic floors and dropped bladders later. Yep. We're going there. Aren't you excited? You might want to pee first before we get there.

2. I Swear I'm Listening, So Why Do I Have to Ask People to Repeat Themselves More Often?

Seriously, is it just me, or have all Boomers damaged their eardrums listening to rock-n-roll? It was an exciting time. Technology was advancing and so was the music industry. Suddenly we could carry our favorite artists' performances around with us. We pumped up the volume on our Walkmans, popped our headphones on, and nothing ever sounded the same again. The music we listened to was changing as much as the delivery system — from the smooth, innocent sounds of Paul Anka and The Righteous Brothers to the raucous anthems of Queen and Kiss. It was all becoming so liberated. Songs were suddenly more than a pretty melody; they were now narratives about life, and often outcries for freedom and change.

These days, however, many Boomers find it difficult to hear what our dinner companions are saying to us, even if we're closely seated at a small table. It's very frustrating; on the other hand, it's quite nice at a wedding where you hardly know anyone.

And who the heck turned the television volume up so loud? Obviously, someone else must have done it. It couldn't have been me. Or was it? Nah, couldn't have been me, had to have been those darn kids.

I always try to look at the positive side of aging. I guess I can accept a little hearing loss if it means I'm not disturbed by the sounds of my husband's snoring at night or my boys yelling at their Fortnite opponents while playing on their Xboxes.

3. I Look the Same. I Really Do. So Why are There Some Features I Just Don't Recognize?

I'm talking about those lines and wrinkles — or worse, those pesky little red and brown spots that suddenly appear out of nowhere. I remember hearing my mom complain about them, preferring to call them *sunspots* but never age spots. And now, here I am counting the speckles on my own skin.

There are hundreds of skincare creams: creams to hydrate, exfoliate, lighten, brighten, and tighten the skin. Don't we all have drawers full of them? I've always taken pristine care of my skin morning and night, but I will admit that I haven't always been as kind to it when it comes to the sun. I love being outdoors and sporting a tan year-round if I can. It is one of my guilty pleasures. But now I know to be super vigilant

41

and always wear sunscreen so I don't burn.

4. I'm Cool with Aging; It's Just That One Thing About it Weighs on Me More Than Others.

While we may be able to hide irregularities on our skin, there's not much we can do to hide the extra pounds that seem to mysteriously appear each passing year. I swear I'm not eating more than before. The fat in our bodies just seems to slyly shift to new places! I can't believe how much my waistline has changed, and not in a good way. It's not that I weigh that much more, it's just that the weight seems to have redistributed itself, so my favorite shorts — the ones I've had forever — just don't button like they used to. And I'm not getting rid of those shorts!

5. If Memory Serves Me Correctly, I Don't Remember Much.

Okay, I know you've been waiting to see if I was going to bring up this one. Wait. What was I talking about again?

Oh, right. Yes, I suffer from CRS, *can't remember s@*t!*

In fact, I don't want to brag, but I can forget what I'm doing while I'm doing it.

I'd like a nickel for every time I ask,

"Where are my glasses?" I swear I lose them ten times a day. The most embarrassing part is that sometimes, after searching my entire house, looking in every conceivable spot where I might have left them, retracing my steps several times, I finally come to the realization that I'm actually wearing them. Oh yeah, there they are, as plain as the nose on my face — the one that's holding up my glasses!

Or I'll reach up and feel a pair on top of my head *while* I am wearing a pair.

When this happens, I really don't know what to do first, laugh or cry. So I laugh — at least for now. Of course, we can't laugh too hard (or sneeze for that matter), for fear we may leak . . . okay, there, I said it.

And can we talk about remembering names for just a minute? With a husband, seven kids, four grandkids, and a dog, I often find myself cycling through a phonebook worth of names before I call the right person down to dinner. I have learned to say "girls and boys" and "ladies and gentlemen" and sometimes just, "Kids, come down and bring the dog."

Do any of you feel like you've lost the ability to recall people's names too? Sometimes even your best friend's. Yikes! I hate when this happens.

I'd like to introduce you to my friend . . . My friend . . . who is a great friend . . . Whom I have known since childhood . . . Please say hello to my friend . . . um . . . I'm sorry. But I've momentarily forgotten her name. Or even worse, "Let me introduce you to my husband . . . I call him 'Honey.' "

Is this a natural aging occurrence? Or is this an early sign of dementia? I personally think that I just hit on the all-time scariest fear that any of us will encounter as we grow older: *forgetfulness.*

6. Can I Take a Pass on Those Senior Passes?

Finally, you know you're aging when you're asked if you would like the senior discount at the movie theater.

Excuse me? What did you just say? Do I *look* like a senior citizen? No, really, let's go into the bathroom so you can look at me in that unforgiving light.

When the day comes that *senior discounts* start arriving in the mail, some people jump for joy just thinking about the money they're going to save, while others want to put their head in the oven. As for me, I'm one of the latter. What made me jump for joy recently was when a young woman *carded me* before scanning a bottle of wine

44

I was purchasing for a dinner party that evening.

"Wait, you want to see my driver's license to check if I'm old enough to buy a bottle of wine? Really?"

She actually made me show it to her. I was so excited that for a moment I thought about kissing her on the lips. Okay, maybe not. But I did ask my daughter to take a picture of me handing over my I.D. to commemorate the moment. And yes, we posted it on Facebook. Wouldn't you? My daughter also asked, "Should we put this on Instagram and Snapchat as well?" To which I replied, "Huh?"

Shortly thereafter I was knocked off my high horse when I was on a call for a media campaign I was working on. I asked what the target audience would be for our outreach and the answer came back, "We're going for seniors, pretty much anyone over 50." Are you kidding me?

So again, all this got me thinking . . . *Is this old age? Have I arrived already?* Sure, I have some of the signs of aging, but I don't feel old. So where does that leave me? I guess it leaves me writing a book about it.

I think about how my mind and my body will wear down with time. Who doesn't? Okay, maybe my teenagers don't, but they will someday. Just as we do. Even more, I think about what I can do to slow that process — what I can do to maintain my body and brain health long into the future.

Don't we all feel that way?

If we're always looking for our glasses or our car keys, isn't our next thought, *Am I already on the road to dementia?* That road is not on my GPS. Pull over, I'm getting out! Sorry life, this is not a road I'm going down willingly.

I know I'm not the only one who has this thought!

I'm also certain I'm not the only one wondering how well I'm doing at the game of aging. Not that I am keeping score, but truly, some people do age better than others. Why is that?

I know worrying about it won't help anything! But talking about it will. In fact, if we don't talk about aging, it will leave each of us feeling like we're dealing with this stage of life alone.

It really is time to start the conversation. Am I right?

By the way, if you just answered, "Hell no, I'm not thinking about any of this right now," I promise you, you will be soon enough. So even if you're not seriously contemplating it at the moment, I hope you'll still read this book so that you get a head start on this whole aging thing. I totally wish someone had given me this playbook when I was in my 40s!

CHAPTER 3
OLD AGE!
ARE WE THERE YET?

"The secret of staying young is
to live honestly, eat slowly and
lie about your age."
— LUCILLE BALL

Like a little kid on a long car ride who incessantly asks her parents, "Are we there yet?" don't we all find ourselves asking the same question about old age?

Do you recall when you first asked yourself this? I know the moment for me. It was a warm September morning. After slipping into a sundress and sandals I gave myself one last look in the mirror and asked, *Is this skirt too short for a woman my age?* I often find myself asking questions like this now. *Am I too old to wear ripped jeans? How about leggings?* This particular morning, the dilemma was top of mind because my 65th birthday was right around the corner and I could hardly believe I was getting dressed to make my way to the Social Security office.

At first, I thought about going incognito. Maybe I'd wear a baseball cap and sunglasses — or one of my wigs from my chemo days. But I didn't. Okay, admittedly I did take my biggest pair of sunglasses!

Like all government offices, when I arrived, they asked me to sign in, take a seat, and wait until they called my name.

What? Honestly at that moment I considered telling her my name was Suzanne Somers but I didn't. Still . . .

Someone is going to call out my name in front of this entire room full of people?!

Oh God, please, I don't want them to shout out my name. Not in this office.

For fifteen minutes, I stood close to the window where the woman who called out names was sitting so she wouldn't have to say mine too loud. I even considered gifting her $100 to whisper my name. Honestly, I've never been more focused on one person — not even when I interviewed Prince Charles.

Finally, it was my turn.

"Ms. Lunden, go to window number eight."

When I sat down in front of the open glass partition, I must have looked like a deer in headlights because the Social Security agent took one look at me and said, "Yeah, I know lady, you just can't believe you're here. You're not alone; I hear it a dozen times a day."

Was it that obvious?

When I was a little girl, I admittedly used to think of 65 as *really* old — as in the-end-of-the-road kind of old. Now, here I am driving full speed through my 60s with the top down and the wind blowing through my hair, feeling like it's one of the best decades of my life. I didn't expect it to be, and that's a shame. We really shouldn't make this wonderful discovery about aging looking in the rearview mirror.

I cringe when I recall my own predictions about this time of life! I mean, my hair isn't gray. (Okay, okay, I've never let my roots grow out long enough to see my natural color and was totally shocked to spy a little silver patch on each temple when it began to grow back after my cancer treatment.) I also don't have trouble getting out of a chair. (Well, most of the time.) I haven't turned in my jeans for golf pants. (Although maybe for some mom jeans.) And I still work out and climb mountains. (They're not quite Mount Elbrus, but some of the hills in Connecticut are pretty steep.)

50

Heck, what I'm saying is, I'm so far from the frail granny I thought I'd be. It's fair to say that most of us 60-somethings look quite different today than the generations that came before us. The character Maude was 47 at the beginning of that eponymous series. The silver-haired Aunt Bea (of *The Andy Griffith Show*) was 58, and the Golden Girls were in their 60s (and Sofia in her 70s) — younger than I am now, but they seemed so much older.

There are a number of things that have kept us from retiring to the sidelines, including better health care, fitness programs, fashions, hairstyles, and cosmetics, to say nothing of Botox and plastic surgery for some. However, there's another critical component that I think has brought us closer to the fountain of youth than any cream in a jar or hair color from a bottle could, and that is our mindset. Having an *expectation* that we will remain healthy, engaged, and full of vitality as we pass through our later decades is a serum all of its own.

People no longer feel compelled to check out at any particular age and shrink into the background. Instead, as we enter our 50s, 60s, and 70s today, we are more inclined to sign up for Zumba classes, marathons, college courses, and travel adventures.

It does seem that while we were in our 30s, 40s, and even our 50s, we thought of ourselves as being *in that decade.* We'd say, "I'm a 30-something" or "I'm a 40-something." And when we were not defining ourselves by decade, we were identified by our generation, saying we were Baby Boomers. Other generations are labeled too. There's the Greatest Generation, the Silent Generation, Generation X, Gen Y or Millennials, and now there's Generation Z, iGen, or Centennials. Those are a lot of labels! But whatever decade or generation we're in, we shouldn't let it affect the way we view our possibilities.

It makes me sad to think that, even if we are vivacious, vibrant, and still flourishing in our careers, when we pass 50 and head for 60, we begin to think of ourselves by how well we are aging. We should be able to define ourselves by how much we live and love life, and not confine ourselves to the decade or age we are presently or the generation into which we were born.

I'm currently approaching my twentieth wedding anniversary with my husband, Jeff Konigsberg, a businessman who owns summer camps for children. One such camp, with a lake, 17 tennis courts, and a climbing wall, is now my summer playground. Jeff is ten years younger than me. We were born a *decade* apart. Yet we've been a perfect match all these years. We're both living incredibly busy lives, always travelling, keeping crazy, demanding work schedules, and still making time for fun. Oh, did I forget to say that Jeff and I also have two sets of teenaged twins in our house?! (You read that right. I said *two* sets of *teenaged twins*.) Yet, despite all this activity, when I think about my life and my health today, I realize that I have succumbed to the societal trap of speaking about it in terms of how I'm doing *for my age*. There's that ugly qualifier again.

By the time you're reading this book, I will be 69. How the heck did that happen? Seriously, the idea that I am going to turn 70 soon just does not seem possible. It's almost as if I've entered *The Twilight Zone.* There is a fifth dimension beyond that which is known to man. It is a dimension as vast as space and as timeless. A dimension where Joan Lunden, a 45-year-old in her own mind, is forced to face the AGE ZONE.

"Inside every older person is a younger person wondering . . . What the f*@*

53

Once this kind of thinking becomes the way we measure our life, we suddenly become much more conscious of the aging process. We begin to take inventory of our physical and mental changes. We make comparisons to our former selves — or worse, to others. This is why it's so important not to give in to the little voice that limits you and leaves you fretting all day instead of doing something fulfilling.

This leads me to another important point. There is one aspect of life that I feel eases up as we begin to age, which is: *how we experience the passage of time.*

When I say this, you may be thinking about how time seems to zoom by at a more rapid speed as you age. It sure feels as if that's what's happening, doesn't it? But here's what I mean by this statement.

I believe time itself is more comfortable at this stage of the game. I used to feel as if I were constantly running a marathon to keep up with a ticking clock. But as I've grown older, I don't feel as if I have to run out the clock at all anymore. I'm still incredibly busy and carry just as many responsibilities as I always have, but I'm more at ease with myself and with life. That serenity may be wisdom, or it may be age. Either way, I like it.

"Be mindful of how you approach time. Watching the clock is not the same as watching the sun rise."
— SOPHIA BEDFORD-PIERCE

This is the stage when we can stop rehashing and obsessing about mistakes we've made. It's an opportunity to wipe the slate clean, to let go of petty squabbles we've fumed over far too long, and to forgive and forget — not only others, but ourselves too. Some good news: the forgetting part is easier now. The forgiving part is truly necessary. Once we can look at where we've been with a sense of appreciation, we can allow ourselves to look toward a future full of new opportunities and options.

Do you ever find yourself fondly reminiscing about the playfulness of your childhood and a life well lived? I do. And, in many ways, I have my photo archive to thank for that.

I recently began a visual reconstruction of my life. I started going through family albums. Yep. I have real photographs and not just images on my phone. Does that make me old? Maybe, but I am so happy to have those family pictures. I think mine is probably the last generation to have those kinds of keepsakes. The baby photos of every generation thereafter were taken on smartphones!

As I sorted through these pictures and tried to remember names and dates, I realized that I had very few relatives left to ask questions of, so that's when I turned to Ancestry.com. You can find amazing details about your family's past with a simple keystroke.

I also found myself turning to Classmates .com to find old (sorry, there's that word again) high school friends who might help me remember people and events from that period in my life as well.

A few years ago, I built an area in our basement where I keep all of my career files, photographs, and videos. One day as I rummaged through that memorabilia from my life and career, I had what I can only describe as an out-of-body experience. As I stood looking around the room, I suddenly felt as if it were spinning in slow motion. I took in the images of all the plaques, awards, keys to various cities, and pictures of me with celebrities and world leaders. My eyes rested first on a piece of the Berlin

Wall that I got as a souvenir while reporting there; then on a nugget from the moon landing I obtained while covering a story from NASA; and finally on a row of helmets from every branch of the armed forces that I collected during my years of shooting military training missions for my primetime series *Behind Closed Doors.* In that moment, as I examined my professional accomplishments, I found that, perhaps for the first time, I was finally giving myself permission to relish and take pride in them.

By anyone's account, my life has been a thrilling ride, but it did go by at such warp speed. When I look back at all the places I've traveled to and all the honors I've received, there are times when I can't even recall being present for some of these amazing moments.

> "Plenty of people miss their
> share of happiness,
> not because they never found it,
> but because they didn't stop to enjoy it."
> — W. FEATHER

It's kind of mind-boggling. Memories of those events should be treasured for a lifetime, yet they had gone by so unbelievably fast that, in many cases, I find it hard to retrieve the details from my memory bank.

Thank goodness for Google and YouTube, where I often turn to gather the information I can't recollect on my own. I'll admit, this is definitely a perk of living a public life. Not only did I get to cover royal weddings and presidential inaugurations, there are pictures and videos of it all. Truth be told, until I started going through this exercise, I had never given much thought to the fact that my entire adult life was so well documented. So, thank you, Google Images, YouTube, and all of you out there who have uploaded hours of GMA images I didn't have in my own archives!

While I know that not everyone has such things as city keys tucked away in their basements or drawers, I'll bet the *keys* to amazing moments in your life are still stored somewhere in your house, perhaps in your attic or basement, an offsite storage unit, or even online.

No matter where your memorabilia resides, I find that revisiting special moments and milestones is important because they reveal — sometimes even to ourselves — what our life is all about. And in the process, it helps change the way we experience the passage of time.

This process of reflection also prompts us to contemplate how satisfied we are with our life so far, and to determine whether we have achieved all that we've wanted. It also helps us plan what else we might like to do in the years still to come.

It provides an opportunity to set a new course for ourselves, to shape our coming years in ways that fulfill our life dreams so that we can create new memories.

CHAPTER 4
STROLLERS, CARS, AND
WHEELCHAIRS!

"Aging is not lost youth but a new stage
of opportunity and strength."
— BETTY FRIEDAN

When I was 52 years old, I welcomed my
first set of twins, Kate and Max, into the
world. Twenty months later our house was
like Noah's ark . . . the kids were coming
two by two. That's when my husband and I
welcomed our second set of twins, Kim and
Jack. Shortly thereafter, we invited a group
of friends over to celebrate our two newest
bundles of joy. The older twins were squeal-
ing with delight and dancing around the
newborns. As some of my girlfriends came
through the front door, they gasped at the
bedlam before them.

"I'm exhausted just looking at this!" they
exclaimed. Some were Type A workaholics
while others were empty nesters who
couldn't fathom what my husband and I

were undertaking.

A few hours earlier I had a local restaurant deliver food for the occasion. The comments from the European staff really sparked my interest because when those French women saw my toddlers romping around, they joyously exclaimed, *"Oh my, you will never grow old!"*

How about that? I think it's profound that two sets of eyes could view the same situation and come to different conclusions. One found it exhausting, while the other saw it as exhilarating. Perception is reality, right? It sure was that day. But the truth is also circumstantial, because there were and still are days when I vacillate between both points of view. Sometimes I feel as though my two sets of twins keep me feeling young and full of life, and on other days I'm completely worn out! It's not unlike the animal kingdom. How many people do you know who have an older dog and get a puppy to make their older dog feel young and reinvigorated? It usually works. Most of the time, the older dog finds the puppy adorable and plays with it even though its ball chasing days seem to be long over but on other days, the senior dog may just "air bite" the pup as if to say, "Hey kid, my hip is acting up; go play alone for a while." In this scenario I'm the older dog, LOL.

But that is also our crazy new world. In past generations, life and aging felt far more predictable. There was a structure to it that few people challenged. As boys became men, they married and went to work to earn the household income. Women had babies in their 20s and then stayed home to care for them. These traditional beliefs were the way society was structured for hundreds of years. There was also a higher rate of alcoholism, heart disease, and death before 70.

Life today simply does not play out like our grandparents' or even our parents' lives did. Current statistics show people are marrying and having children much later. Perhaps not as late as me, but parents are definitely skewing older. It has also become much more common, if not necessary, for both spouses to hold down jobs while still managing those homes and raising their families.

Most young couples have the expectation of living longer, and so do their parents. With this new lifestyle and this evolving aging landscape, there are myriad social, economic, and emotional stresses that come into play.

When our grandparents' generation approached their 50s, their parents had likely passed away and their children were grown and already out on their own. Those generations were considered over-the-hill by age 50, retired by 60, and likely six feet under by 70.

I always got the sense, even from my parents, that you had to have *made it* by the time you were 50. For whatever reason, that age served as a professional benchmark. Your career might extend into your 60s, but until recently, your 60s were generally your retirement years. Basically, 65 was your *use-by* date. When my mom was a young woman starting a family, she didn't anticipate living past 70. She was shocked to make it to almost 95. She told me this repeatedly, especially in her later years.

There wasn't a thought that when a person reached their 50s or 60s, they could find themselves taking care of their older parents while simultaneously still caring for their children. But today our lives and our aging timelines are completely different. There are tens of millions of people who are at some stage of parenting while caring for aging parents. Our generation often finds itself needing to meet demands at both ends of the life spectrum — the needs of our children at one end and the needs of our aging parents on the other.

That is how we became the *Sandwich Generation,* and the challenges certainly require a new playbook. I am part of that generation. In fact, if you look up the term online, you may well find my face staring back at you.

The Challenges of the Sandwich Generation

As it happened during this phase of life, I was changing my twins' diapers at the same time as I was managing the care of my aging mother. My life was controlled bedlam at times (it still is sometimes!), and it's not really where I expected to be in my 50s, yet that was my life and I was loving every minute of it.

At bath time my husband and I would put all four little ones in the tub together. What a bubbly, giggly, sudsy scene that was! We would then have four towels laid laid out on the carpet in the playroom, followed by four diapers, four sets of jammies, and all the tubes of Desitin and baby lotion we needed. It was practically an assembly line!

It baffled me to think that I was picking out strollers — make that double strollers, for Max, Kate, Kim and Jack — while I was also buying cars for my teenaged girls Jamie, Lindsay, and Sarah, and a wheelchair for my mom, Glady.

I took over the care and responsibility of my mother at a young age, much younger than I ever expected. I became financially responsible for her when I was in my early 30s. At first, it was really more like being her personal travel agent. I was fortunate enough to be able to send her on trips all over the world, and she relished every moment of those adventures. I always got such a kick out of her excitement as we planned what she'd see, where she'd eat, and where she'd shop in every foreign city. No doubt, there were times when I'd get a little tired of her first-class travel requests, but she truly enjoyed these jaunts, so I never said no.

Mom was known as *Glitzy Glady,* not just for her effervescent personality but also because of her love of gold purses, gold cowboy boots, gold lamé, and, well, anything else trimmed in gold. It all went so well with her glamorous red hair, which she had until the day she passed away. In fact, one of her famous mottos was, "You dye until you die." I'm with her on that one.

One of the beautiful things about our parents growing older is that they can share with us what they learn about the aging process, and often these can be powerful nuggets of wisdom, hope, and, in the case of my mom, humor. For example, she always enjoyed telling people that she was five years older than she really was; that way, they would tell her, "Oh my, you look so young for your age." My mom never could resist a compliment!

Aging parents also tend to talk about their younger lives since those are the deeply imbedded memories they can most easily tap into. If we are open to listening, we can often glean a lot about our family history and about our parent as a person. I consider this privileged and prized information. You don't have to be a parent to pass on your life experiences. One of my single friends (53 years old, has never been married nor had children) told her eldest niece as she went off to college, "You will make mistakes and bad choices; that is inevitable. But if I have anything to do with it, you won't make *my* mistakes and bad choices." She then handed the young woman a journal. She had been keeping the journal for about ten years, which contained little anecdotes, notes of wisdom, and stories that she had collected with the sole reason to be a gift to her nieces. She wanted them to have her perspective as a single woman living in NYC. *Everyone* is important in passing on family legacy.

66

CAPTURING YOUR FAMILY STORY

Choose a time and a location that will make your family member feel comfortable. Set up your video camera or iPhone to record somewhere where you'll have good sound quality. The most important thing to capture is their voices — their audio stories. Construct an interview list ahead of time.

Childhood/Family Life
- Do you know the story of your birth?
- What is the origin of your name?
- Where did you grow up? What was it like there? (big city, small town, rural area?)
- What was the world like when you were growing up? What were your family's greatest concerns? (peace, war, recession?)
- What were you like as a child? (sensitive, rambunctious, defiant, class clown?)
- Can you tell me about your parents and siblings?
- Tell me about your education throughout your life.

Adult Life

- Tell me about your professional career. Was it what you expected it to be?
- How did you and Mom/Dad meet and marry? (if it's a parent)
- What do admire most about your spouse?
- What accomplishments are you the proudest of?

Parenthood

- What was the world like when I was a child?
- What was I like as a child?
- What are the biggest differences between the way you raised us and the way we raise kids today?

Family History

- Do we have any famous/infamous family members?
- Are there any family scandals that are too good not to tell?
- Are there any chronic illnesses that we should know about? (What is it? Who had it? What were the ages at which people got diagnosed?)

Philosophical/Fun Questions
- What are your best qualities? Worst qualities?
- Do you have any favorite sayings or expressions?
- If you could go back to any age, which would it be and why?
- If you won $1 million tomorrow, what would you do with the money?
- Do you have a philosophy on life? What's your best piece of advice for living and aging?

The Present and the Future
- What brings you the most pleasure today?
- How are you dealing with the aging process? What have been the best/worst/hardest parts?
- Do you have a bucket list? What's on it?
- How do you envision your life in the coming years? If there comes a time when you can no longer live safely on your own, where would you like to live?

- Do you have the following documents: Will, Living Will, Durable Power of Attorney, Health care Power of Attorney/Health Care Proxy, DNR/DNI, Advanced Health Care Directive?
- Do you have any special requests for your Bon Voyage party? (their funeral)
- What do you want people to remember about you?

You'll likely get some fascinating answers. This kind of video recording of your family history is priceless.

My mom was an eternal optimist! She taught me to reach for the stars and to expect great things both of myself and of life. Move over Eckhart Tolle, my mom was my original guru of positive thinking.

Through her perspective, I learned some of the most valuable lessons in life. She definitely inspired me to be an independent young woman who dared to venture into a man's field — the television news business — and to make my way up the ladder.

When I was 25 and anchoring the news in

my hometown of Sacramento, I invited my mom to have lunch one day after the noon broadcast. She was super proud that my television career was taking off; she never missed one of my broadcasts. However, the reason I'd invited her to lunch that afternoon was to tell her that I had received an exciting job offer from the ABC TV affiliate in New York City. They wanted me to be a field reporter and the weekend anchor. The offer meant I would be leaving my local TV job and moving to the Big Apple — one of the largest markets in television. This was a huge opportunity for me. I wanted and needed my mom's support.

I watched her expression vacillate between excitement for me and disappointment for her. Although I would make it a priority to return home to see her often, she'd no longer be able to watch me on TV every day as she always had. Once she absorbed the news, she enthusiastically said, "Joni, while I hate the idea of not having you here with me, I know that you are destined to do big things. I can see your name in lights, so you just keep shooting for the stars and don't ever doubt that you can make it to the top."

In typical mom fashion, she had just the right words at the right time. Hearing her positive affirmations were incredibly impactful throughout my life. They inspired and motivated me to always follow my dreams. In case you can't tell, my mom was a real spitfire. But even women as vivacious and excited about life as she was can hit a point when they must put down their travel guides and pick up the *TV Guide* instead. It was a difficult transition to witness. Her decline was slow, but noticeable.

As Mom grew older, I watched her check out. Her life of leisure travel and social parties was over. She folded up her St. John pant suits, put away her gold heels, and seemingly settled in for old age. Like millions of others, I became her caregiver almost overnight.

About the same time my mom was slowing down, my brother, Jeff, also needed to be cared for. He was suffering from many of the debilitating complications of Type II diabetes. We all decided that it would be best if I moved my mom and my brother into a condominium together. I arranged for an aide to help them a few days a week. They were very comfortable and happy living that way and came to depend on each other.

As their health declined, my mom and I often discussed their living situation. She wanted to move to an active senior community like all of her friends had done. We'd even visited some of the communities where these friends were living. They, too, were encouraging her to make the move — everyone loved having vivacious Glady around.

In retrospect, I wish I had been more persistent about moving her there while she was in her 70s. She would have played robust card games, gone shopping with her girlfriends, and spent evenings at the movies or participating in other fun social events. They would have laughed and made lots of new memories together.

Mom knew deep down that she would enjoy living that life and that it would keep her feeling young and vibrant, but she wouldn't leave my brother. He was unable to move to the senior community because he smoked cigarettes, something they didn't allow. My brother's smoking habit created a real conundrum. He couldn't or wouldn't stop. He was in his mid-50s and was battling so many serious health issues that I sometimes wonder if smoking was the only thing he could still enjoy.

Over time, as their health declined, so did their outside social connections and engagements. My brother's diabetes progressed to the point where he was sometimes too sick to even leave his room, so Mom went from living with a close companion to being a recluse with no one to talk to.

While my mom wasn't living alone, she was experiencing bouts of loneliness. She had none of the stimulation, conversation, and sense of the security she had once enjoyed when the two of them cooked, watched TV together, and talked for hours about life. Eventually, the combination of smoking and diabetes contributed to Jeff's death at an early age.

Living that way ultimately robbed my mom of much of her wellness and happiness, especially in her later years, and it seemed, at least to me, to exponentially accelerate her dementia.

When I looked into this theory of mine, I found that loneliness raises our stress hormone levels and causes inflammation associated with a wide range of health issues. It can lead to a higher risk of heart attack, stroke, anxiety, depression, and dementia. Social isolation is also thought to be on a par with high blood pressure, obesity, lack of exercise, and smoking as a risk factor for early death.

Researchers at Brigham Young University have found that isolation and loneliness are as detrimental to our health as smoking fifteen cigarettes a day, and that lonely people are fifty percent more likely to die prematurely than those with healthy social relationships.

Managing our parents' later years doesn't always go as smoothly as we'd like. I have long regretted that I let my mother *check out* as she did. I felt like her life shouldn't have come to a screeching halt like that. But knowing what I know now, I think what may have been happening was the dementia had started to take over her world. She no longer felt confident galivanting around and putting herself in unfamiliar airports and hotels. I'll admit, I get that.

My mom seemed to stop running the bases just like that. She turned in her uniform and forfeited the rest of the game. I don't think it was a conscious move on her part, but it was very apparent to me and to all of her friends.

"Years may wrinkle the skin, but to give up enthusiasm wrinkles the soul."
— SAMUEL ULLMAN

My mom's gradual retreat from life and slide into dementia broke my heart. Could I have put my foot down for her sake? Maybe.

I've certainly asked myself that question many times. I think many of us grapple with these types of nagging questions as we help our parents navigate their later years. One thing is for sure, though, being a part of my mom's aging journey made me really think about my own.

It felt like Glitzy Glady's spark had been extinguished. Would that happen to me? I certainly don't want to believe that my fire will go out like that.

Oh no, I want to stay in this game of life as long as possible. I see myself racing around third base slightly out of breath, digging down deep to grasp one last blast of air and adrenalin, then wildly sliding face-first into home base sending dirt flying all over the place while the crowd cheers, "What an amazing run, Lunden!" With all my children at the dugout high-fiving one another, taking pictures, and remembering that their mother's life had been a splendid home run!

CHAPTER 5
I'M NOT OLD; I'M 45 PLUS
SHIPPING AND HANDLING

"There's no such thing as anti-aging.
We're all aging, period. Women take it as
something personal that they are getting
older. They think that they failed
somehow by not staying 25. This is crazy
to me because my belief is that it's a
privilege to get older — not everybody
gets to get older."

— CAMERON DIAZ

Remember the 1960s when kids on college campuses who were opposed to the Vietnam War chanted, "Hell no, we won't go!" Well, those college kids are today's Boomers *in* their 60s (or older) and they're still chanting, "Hell no, we won't go!" This time, of course, they are resisting being drafted into old age. The Boomer generation has always been defined by its tendency to push back, so it shouldn't really surprise anyone that they're pushing back again and refusing to grow old.

The Boomers' new call to action is: "Change the rules of aging." Or, as I once heard, "Don't let age change you, change the way you age!"

There are 75 million Boomers in this country. Every 8 seconds one of them turns 65. As Boomers have made their way through the decades, they've seemed determined to reshape the concept of aging. I think we've done a pretty good job of it — but there's still room for improvement.

Just because there's a silver tsunami of Boomers signing up for Social Security doesn't mean they are willing to sign up for *old age.* The National Council on Aging conducted a nationwide survey of people between the ages of 65 to 72. The survey found that Boomers simply were not willing to call themselves "middle-aged." In fact, half of them described themselves as young! Most said that old age begins at 70 for a man and, 75 for a woman.

When a massive generation defies the stereotypes, rewrites the rules, and refuses to give up physically or adopt an old mindset, they have basically redefined the stages of life as we've known them.

The once passive Golden Years have been replaced by a new active *Third Age,* which is generally understood to be that span of time between retirement and the beginning of age-imposed physical and cognitive limitations. In today's world this Third Age occurs roughly between the ages of 65 to 80 and can even extend further for some people.

The first time I ever heard the term Third Age was when I was asked to do an interview with a website called ThirdAge. com. When I inquired about the meaning of the website's name, the writer told me that this period represents that stage of life when people are retired from work but not retired from life. I loved that! She said their website specialized in information for those who had arrived at this stage that is both old age yet not old age.

I was intrigued by this concept so much that I began researching its origins. I found that the term Third Age was first proposed in the 1980s through a book titled *A Fresh Map of Life: The Emergence of the Third Age* by Peter Laslett, a British historian. According to Laslett, one's life consists of four ages. The First Age is a period of dependence, socialization, and learning; the Second Age is a period of independence, working, and childrearing; the Third Age is a period of life fulfillment; and then, when one declines in health and/or cognitive function, they enter the Fourth Age, which is essentially an era of frailty and dependence.

Laslett predicted that the Third Age would only emerge in developed countries where retired people have sufficient funds from pensions and savings to live out this extended stage of life. He attributed the following characteristics to people in their Third Age:

- Being mentally and physically healthy
- Being able to enjoy an active social life
- Having time to find fulfilment

It turns out Laslett's 1980s theory proved to be true, for his Third Age has certainly taken hold in the United States. Today's longevity experts know much more about how our brain functions and what aspects of human behavior keep our spirit alive and well. These are the top predictors they cite for successfully navigating this new extended life stage:

- Staying engaged in life
- Maintaining meaningful social relationships
- Continuing to learn
- Having a sense of purpose

When we are interested and passionate about something in life, it gives us a reason to wake up in the morning and get excited for the day. If we want to consciously age well, it is critical that we all have an understanding of the factors that will give us our best chance at health and happiness during those extra years.

I, for one, want to be part of this new Third Age as I get older, and I want to be prepared to enjoy it. But it does take some thought and planning. Seemingly, while this Third Age emerged and changed the rules of aging, it happened without most people noticing. Consequently, a lot of people are finding themselves facing their later years unprepared.

Here are some of the questions we need to be exploring to be ready for our Third Age.

- What kind of lifestyle do I want?
- Do I wish to find an active senior community or remain in my home?
- Am I nurturing friendships so I'll continue to have meaningful connections?
- Are there things I'd like to do to help others so I have a sense of purpose?
- What will I be doing to challenge my

brain so I can retain my cognitive abilities?

- Do I have my stress under control, so I am able to enjoy inner peace as I age?
- Am I making healthy life choices so that I will be able to maintain my health?
- Am I taking steps to ensure that I won't be a burden to my family?

My husband and I are having these kinds of discussions about how we want our lives to look as we age. They are not morose discussions; they are fun and exciting, because that is the way we are choosing to approach our Third Age.

We often laugh about some of our Third Age requirements: a warm sunny climate for golf and pool time; an active community where we can maintain our fitness and also remain socially connected; a one-story living space that doesn't require climbing any stairs in case our bodies start to fall apart; at least two big screen TVs so I can watch crime-scene dramas while he watches basketball and mixed martial arts cage fighting; and last, but not least, a place that is small enough so it doesn't require much upkeep but is also big enough for our kids to visit.

I said visit. *Not* live with us.

What excites you?

What makes you bounce out of bed to get your day started?

For me, these days it's continuing to have the opportunity to use my skills and platform to inform and empower others in the field of health and wellness, whether through media campaigns, public speaking engagements, or day-to-day interactions with my peer group.

I relish the opportunity to speak to people all over the country. I love everything about it, from writing the speeches and travelling, to mingling and shaking hands with attendees. There's no better way to hear what people want and need than to engage them in meaningful and purposeful conversation. That's one of the reasons I enjoy doing meet and greets before or after an event. It keeps me current and connected. And of course, I continue to be excited to have the opportunity to wake up and still write books.

On a personal level, I'm thrilled to attend my kids' basketball, soccer, and football games. I've become a genuine sports fan, though I will admit that I sometimes get a little carried away and can be a bit too vocal in the stands — at least that's what the kids say. My husband is there, though, to keep me in check. Finally, I'm always excited to get back to whatever book I am reading. It seems like I've fallen in love with reading all over again. I used to *have* to read for work, but now I savor each story and its characters, and I allow myself to be swept away to another time and place, living in the characters' world for a brief time. As I grow older, being able to immerse myself in books even more is one thing I am really looking forward to as my workload diminishes.

Each of us needs to give some thought to what makes us happy in life, especially now that we will likely have a whole lot of time for such pursuits. Because to live the life you want going forward, you need a plan.

So, what do you want your future to look like?

In life and aging, strategy matters! With a plan in hand, we're more apt to embrace these years than we are to try to dodge them. What's holding you back? Begin making a list of what you want your future to look like.

As we age, many people find that they can finally pursue passion projects they never had time for before. Maybe you always wanted to volunteer to help children, animals, or members of your community, but you were too busy working. Or maybe you've been yearning to travel but had to tend to too many things in *your* world to actually see *the rest of the world.*

At first, the idea of finding things to fill our days can be daunting. But that feeling doesn't usually last very long. I know a lot of people who are finally pursuing passions, such as photography and painting, and immensely enjoying them!

I've often thought about going back to school. I'd love to enroll in some college classes. I'd be interested in courses on health and nutrition. I know; what a shock, right? As a past psychology and sociology major, I'm always intrigued to learn more about other societies and the people who live there. There is so much happening in our world today. How is the rest of the world faring? How is life changing in other parts of the world as job markets shift away from farming and manufacturing and technology takes even greater precedence? I may have to get busy writing a college essay to get into the school of my choice. Do you think my family will mind moving so I can be near campus?

It's not unusual for people to head back to the classroom as they age. It's even having an effect on the industry of senior living. There is a growing number of senior communities being built next to and in partnership with universities so that senior residents can take part in college life. They take classes; attend sports, theatre, and music events as well as lectures; and even eat in the campus dining hall. This new concept gives seniors an opportunity to continue learning and to stay socially active with an even younger, energetic age group. It seems to me like a win-win proposition.

Even if you hated school and couldn't wait to graduate when you were in college, this is a different time in life when it could be fun to learn something new just because it interests you. You can always audit classes. By that I mean attend, listen to, learn from, and enjoy them without being tested or graded. Oh yeah, now we're talking! Now, that's a perk of aging!

Whatever our dreams may be, the Third Age holds infinite possibilities for us to grow, feel relevant, *and* have fun. I hear from two types of people on social media: those who are idle and don't know what to do with their time and those who are busy enjoying their newfound freedoms. I have found that the difference between the two is often as simple as having a plan.

I have to share one story that I especially loved. A very lively and spirited woman in her early 60s wrote to tell me that she had worked her whole life for her local utility company as one of the *linemen*. I looked that term up and saw that it's a person who is trained to install, maintain, and repair the high-power lines that deliver our electrical power. Okay, so can we just all agree that's an unbelievably unique job for a woman to have held her whole life?

The woman told me that when she's not working on a power line, she's attending college classes to become an EMT (Emergency Medical Technician), so that she can start an *encore* career when she retires from the utility company. She wasn't lamenting that she'd have to keep working. Quite the contrary, she was excited about her new opportunity! I really love this lady and her fierce determination. Not only did she plan her future, she's taking it by storm!

What are you doing to take your future by storm? Are you a light drizzle, gently watering your Third Stage of life? Or are you a full tsunami, tearing apart beliefs of what you should be and getting ready to rebuild?

Let's all start planning so that we'll be ready to live and thrive in this redefined next chapter of life called the Third Age.

CHAPTER 6
NOT ONLY IS MY SHORT-TERM MEMORY BAD, SO IS MY SHORT-TERM MEMORY

"I've learned two important lessons in life. I can't recall the first one, but the second is that I need to start writing things down."
— UNKNOWN

It's time to address the elephant in the room.

Oh wait, it's only me here in the room.

Just standing and wondering, *Why did I come into this room?*

Has this ever happened to you? You leave one room and walk into another only to find yourself thinking, *Hmmm, I know I came in here for a reason.*

How about when you're looking all over your house for your car keys? You search your purse . . . where did you put them? Obviously not where you usually leave them. Think about the pants you were wearing or the jacket you had on — did either have pockets? Ugh, do I have to go through my laundry basket again?

Then there's this worrisome slip of the mind: You park your car; turn off the ignition; gather your purse, keys, and sunglasses; open the door; and try to get out. What the heck? Oops, good luck exiting with your seatbelt still on. I can't confirm or deny this has ever happened to me. Just saying.

How about when you can't even find your car in a parking lot. No, I'm not joking; I'm really serious. Have you ever walked out of a mall, looked out over the vast sea of cars, and felt a wave of panic come over you — even if just for a few seconds — because you couldn't remember where you parked? I've actually taken to snapping a picture of the marker nearest my car, just in case.

Do these moments send a chill through your body? Stir a sense of dread even?

I know I am not alone. People tell me all sorts of stories about their increasing forgetfulness. I've heard everything from finding scissors in the freezer without any logical explanation for why they're there, to a couple placing purple light bulbs in the sconces outside their front door so they could always find their home at night. Oy vey!

I actually googled how to find my wallet once and discovered that there's an app for that! *Of course* there is. It seems like there's an app for everything these days. Within seconds I downloaded it, so it must be a fairly common occurrence. Phew! Now, don't you feel better too?

I know I do.

While our children might be humored by these now near-daily absentmindedness, if you're like me, as soon as you experience one of these moments, a horrifying fear pulses through your veins like a bolt of electricity. It's the fear of how aging is affecting your brain. Usually I find that if I wait the mental fog out for a few minutes, or do another task, the intended reason for being in that room will eventually come back to me.

Of all the aging fears, I think forgetfulness is the most concerning issue for most of us. What is it that causes cognitive decline, and what can we do to try to avoid it? The good news is, there is a lot of research in this field and much progress is being made. The bad news is, sometimes it just happens.

The human brain is an incredible masterpiece — an example of exquisite engineering. By the time we are born, it has developed more than 100 billion neurons (microscopic cells with teeny-tiny branches that veer off into different directions), and those neurons will be connected by trillions of active synapses so the brain can ultimately communicate with the whole body.

This miraculous organ begins to form just three weeks after conception. By the fifth week, the first synapses are already sending rapid-fire messages to neurons in the fetus's developing limbs.

Then, somewhere between the sixteenth and twentieth week of pregnancy, an ultrasound reveals the fetus's almost fully matured brainstem, which ultimately controls our breathing and heart rate. From this point on, the brain's development really accelerates. A myelin sheath coats the nerves enabling them to communicate at hyper speed. It's as if a WIFI extender is installed to boost signals throughout the human ethernet.

During the first years of life, the brain continues to grow, forming as many as one million neural connections every second! A toddler's brain, astonishingly enough, is already roughly 80 percent the size of an adults. Would you look at the brain on Junior?!

Throughout our tween years, our personality and many of our intellectual faculties take shape. Children test and evolve their social skills. During this time, the brain also begins a grooming process called *synaptic pruning* where it eliminates any of the synapses that are not being used frequently enough to maintain their strength. This allows the whole neural network to function at its best.

By our teenage years our brain reaches its full size, though skills such as impulse control, cognitive reasoning, risk assessment, and judgement still have a long journey to completion. Full development may not occur for some until our mid-thirties. I guess that would explain a lot of the ridiculously dumb things I did in my teens and twenties. And if you think I'm going to 'fess up to those moronic moves, think again. But I blame my brain for all of it.

Would you be surprised to learn that our brain undergoes more changes in our lifetime than any other part of our body? It does. Just like our muscles, parts of it can shrink when underutilized. As it happens, only the hippocampus — the part responsible for memory and learning — shrinks. Although you might think that happens around age 60, the truth is it can and often does occur as early as our 20s, though I suspect few people notice because they haven't been conditioned to fear memory decline the way those of us our age have been!

It is believed that we lose one percent of our hippocampuses' volume annually.

By our 30s our communication skills slow down as does our ability to think. Simply put, we aren't quite as sharp as we were when we were studying for (and quite possible acing) the SAT and GMAT. The result: you guessed it. We suddenly find ourselves searching for a person's name — and I'm not talking about historical figures here, I'm talking about the names of people we know.

From our mid-40s to 50s we may find it more difficult to learn new things. While I've been a bit of a Debbie Downer in these last few paragraphs, let me tell you something positive about our brain at this stage of life. During these latter years, we see an increase in our ability to read social situations and to better control our emotions. We become a better people person. That's a silver lining to look forward to, right?

By our 60s, after a lifetime of gathering knowledge, accessing that information can feel like a stretch. What's up with that? It's taken half a decade or more to accumulate this information and now we can't seem to recall it? Worse, that blank slate leaves a lot of us just a little bit worried that we may be experiencing the beginning of dementia. Luckily for most of us though, that's not the case. Still, it can be scary.

To be clear, while aging can have a negative effect on our memory, it is not necessarily indicative of a problem. As I said, it's normal for younger people to experience memory loss too. They just don't stress or obsess about it, much less notice it. How many times have you asked your teenaged child where they dropped their shoes? Or even schoolbooks? Only to hear, "Uh, I dunno"?

However, in our 70s and 80s, the risk for developing Alzheimer's begins to increase. It can be as high as fifty percent by the time we are 85. Researchers don't yet know why the risk jumps so dramatically then. They suspect it may be linked to inflammation, another natural part of aging, which can lead to a build-up of deposits in the hippocampus — again, that part of the brain responsible for memory. But make no mistake, it is our lifestyle habits that contribute to the majority of our risks for Alzheimer's and dementia.

At the University of California, Davis, researchers found four factors contributed to faster declines in brain volume and brain health: high blood pressure, diabetes, cigarette smoking, and being overweight or obese. Midlife obesity is thought to accelerate brain aging by 10 years.

Other factors include sugar and alcohol consumption. Of course, sugar seems to consciously and subconsciously find its way into all of our diets. Think you'll solve the problem by drinking diet soda instead? Well, I hate to tell you that these beverages are listed as agents of brain aging, too, particularly because of their adverse effect on the hippocampus. Remember, that's the part of the brain that makes and recalls memories . . . just in case you've forgotten.

Studies also indicate that taking care of your heart is another way to effectively care for your brain. It's important to regularly check and treat high blood pressure and high cholesterol. Vigilance in these matters can make a big difference.

Here's the good news from the brain brainiacs researching this challenge — there are lifestyle choices we can make to help retain our short-term memory and keep us as sharp as a person who is decades younger. Now we're talking. I'm in. Are you?

Bear in mind, though, that these improvements won't just magically occur. If we do nothing to change our habits, a number of our mental skills will naturally begin to slow down over time. Even if we are healthy, we can't stop our brains from changing with age.

So what are the behaviors and the lifestyle choices that experts agree will help protect our brains from aging? Following are some easy steps we can all take to stay as mentally agile as possible.

Break a Sweat

Exercise is at the top of the list because it can slow or even reverse the brain's physical decline the way it does with our muscles. When we are physically active, blood is pumped to the brain along with essential nutrients, literally helping to build new brain cells.

For years, scientists thought that we were all born with a set number of brain cells and that we never generated any more. However, in the 1990s, new brain research revealed that a process called *neurogenesis* can and does occur throughout our lives. Neurogenesis, as the name implies, is the creation of new brain cells. And it's now believed that exercise jump-starts that process.

What's more, you can bulk up your brain the same way you can bulk up your muscles. One of the most promising findings in this

96

area of research is the effect that exercise has, not just on the creation of these cells, but on their functionality as well. Brain cells can only improve our intellect if they can connect with the existing neural network. When they are unable to do so, they eventually die. Scientists have long understood that learning something new can create new neurons, but those new neurons only serve us when they are hooked up properly. Neurons created by exercising seem to be more adept at linking up to the neural network. So it looks like exercising is a no-brainer . . . or should I say a *pro-brainer?*

Researchers don't fully understand exactly how exercise affects our minds on a molecular level, but studies show that aerobic exercise is one of the most effective ways to slow the process of brain aging. When combined with resistance exercise on as many days of the week as possible, the two have been found to pack a powerful punch, significantly boosting the brain power of people in the 50-plus age set.

That being said, you don't have to spend hours at the gym to achieve positive results. Walking or cycling for just 30 minutes a day is enough aerobic exercise to reduce brain cell loss. And don't forget, aerobic activity can also significantly reduce the risk of heart attack, stroke, diabetes, and more.

Challenge Your Brain

Along with physical exercise, mental stimulation can work wonders too. Brain experts
tell us that taking a course in an area we've
never studied before, learning a musical
instrument we've never played, or studying
a foreign language we've only dreamed of
speaking can help protect the cognitive
abilities we do have. What's your thinking
activity of choice? It's okay if it's tackling
jigsaw, crossword, or Sudoku puzzles or
quiet leisurely reading . . . it all counts. Even
painting, sculpture, gardening, or chess
playing. What do you think my family would
say if I decided to take up the drums? I
could always get them noise-canceling
headphones! It won't bother me; I told you
earlier I'm not hearing as well as I used to.

It has long been suggested that changing
up simple everyday tasks like brushing our
teeth or combing our hair with our non-
dominant hand can strengthen neural connections in our brain and even grow new
ones. Of course, our hair may look pretty
weird. That being said, it's important to
know that I could not find a lot of hard
evidence to support the importance of these
efforts in protecting our cognitive thinking.

Listen to Music

I read the most fascinating article in a journal called *Neuron.* It shared findings from a study on how listening to music affects the brain. Apparently, doing so can sharpen our ability to anticipate events and stay focused. In the study, researchers took MRIs of people's brains while they were listening to symphonic music and when they were not. An examination of these MRIs showed that the areas of the brain involved with paying attention, making predictions, and accessing memories became very engaged during listening sessions, whereas they did not during those sessions without music.

Not surprisingly, immediately after I read this article I put on my headphones, listened for a while to the songs on my playlist, and soon realized that I was doing all those things they found in the study. Some songs brought back memories, and in order to sing along I had to be able to predict what was coming next. Personally, I love music and I really appreciate a powerful bass, that thundering undercurrent that holds the beat. Yes, I'd love to be a rocker in my next life! But in this one, I'm not that talented or cool.

"When it comes to aging,
we're held to a different standard than men.
A guy said to me: 'Don't you think you're
too old to sing rock n' roll?' I said: 'You'd
better check with Mick Jagger.' "

— CHER

Go Cher!! Turn back time, girl!

Read More

My favorite hobby is reading. My husband's grandmother, Rosie, who passed away just a month shy of her 100th birthday, was a voracious reader. She used to tell me that it was one of the most important things she did for herself. She explained that reading never let her life get boring. She had this saying that I love, "A reader never goes to bed alone." I couldn't agree with her more. If you aren't an avid reader, I highly recommend that you become one. Pick up a book, join a book club, or start listening to audio books. I can't emphasize this enough. In fact, read my lips on this one: READ. MORE. BOOKS. You won't regret it.

Keep Your Cool

Managing stress is important at every stage of life, but especially ours. Whenever we stress out, our brain releases the hormones cortisol and adrenaline. Under certain circumstances, these hormones can be harmful. Because the brain's ability to regulate hormone levels diminishes over time, stress poses greater challenges for us as we age. And chronic stress is particularly damaging as it can kill brain cells, not just reduce their power. While certain kinds of stress are unanticipated, others are very predictable. To help give you more control over the predictable kind, spend some time thinking about and pinpointing the most common triggers, then devise ways to avoid, minimize, or effectively deal with them in advance. Having a plan in place can certainly make life a lot more manageable.

Nurture Relationships

Many of us have saved up for this time in life in the hope that we could live out our years comfortably. We sought wise financial advisors. Some of those advisors said to invest in stocks. Others suggested bonds. Some were more specific, recommending individual bonds over bond funds. It got confusing at times. But here's my very direct investment advice for those of us planning for a long, happy, and healthy life: Invest in *people* bonds. That's right — *invest in bonds with friends, family, and acquaintances.* The return on investment is too great to be fully measured, though scientists have tried, and here is what they've found: Ongoing interaction with others is absolutely necessary to maintain your cognitive abilities. Being socially active not only staves off boredom, it strengthens your focus and attention span, exercises your memory skills, and builds new memories too.

Research from the Assisted Living Federation of America found that when seniors regularly engaged in activities with others, they were more likely to live well into their 90s. According to these studies, good company and the stimulation that ensues can help one live 5.4 years longer on average than those who are less sociable. So phone a friend. Get together. Live longer. Live better.

When you do spend time with others, be sure to plan some fun physical and mental activities. Further studies show that, we are more likely to keep dementia at bay when social interaction is combined with these other pursuits. For example, I love to dance. Thankfully, so do some of my girlfriends whom I work out with. So we added dance, everything from hip-hop to line dancing, to keep exercise fun. We swing with the music and laugh out loud while keeping our blood circulating, our muscles flexing, and our mind busy learning tricky new steps. Who else is ready to boogie down with me?!

Eat Wisely

We all know that eating healthily is good for our fitness and for our heart, but it's also good for our brain. Our brain needs nourishment just like our heart, bones, and muscles, kidneys, liver, and other organs do.

So what are the perfect brain foods? Researchers at Rush University in Chicago studying the association between diet and dementia tell us that older adults should try to follow what they call the MIND diet. It is closest in nature to the Mediterranean diet in that it includes nutrient-rich berries, fruits, and vegetables — especially leafy greens. All of these foods are valued for their antioxidant and anti-inflammatory properties. Add olive oil, nuts, beans, fish, poultry, and whole grains to the shopping list too. Notice that this diet minimizes red meat, dairy, and fried foods to lower the risk of developing Alzheimer's, heart disease, and stroke. Giving proper thought to your diet helps feed the brain!

Get Detoxifying Zzz's

If you want to maintain a beautiful mind, you'll need to get your beauty rest! According to researchers at Duke-NUS, the less older adults sleep, the faster their brains age.

Poor quality or reduced amounts of sleep may be linked to a buildup of beta-amyloid protein in the brain. When this protein clumps together, plaques are formed. These beta-amyloid plaques are a sign of Alzheimer's disease.

According to the Alzheimer Association, the plaques may block cell-to-cell signaling at the synapses. This, in turn, may activate our immune system cells, which can trigger inflammation that is said to devour disabled cells. but can sometimes cause damage to healthy cells too.

There's been a lot of research recently that suggests that during quality sleep, amyloid is cleared from the brain. Neuroscientists at NYU Langone Health's Alzheimer Disease Center in New York City say that this suggests that the better we sleep, the better we clear amyloid from our brain, and that poor sleep may retain amyloid in the brain and therefore lead to Alzheimer's disease. So we need to turn out that light and go to sleep, because quality deep sleep is like a washing machine for our brain.

Be a Light Drinker

I should probably tell you at the outset that I've never been much of a drinker, so I'm certainly not the authority on this one. However, the experts have quite a lot to say on this topic. Have you heard that drinking alcohol sparingly may actually be beneficial to our brains? Several studies have linked having one drink a day for women and two for men with a reduced risk of dementia in older adults. So go ahead, pour yourself a glass of wine, and toast to your health! But don't get carried away — heavy alcohol consumption can do the exact opposite, leading to dementia and the very decline in cognition you were hoping to avoid!

Don't Smoke

In addition to how bad smoking is for your lungs, smoking can affect your body's ability to deliver oxygen and nutrients to the brain and can speed up the brain's natural aging process. Smoking can also lead to the formation of plaques, which can contribute to dementia. When the smoke finally clears, I'm certain you'll see and feel the difference following this advice can make.

Protect Your Head

Extensive research has been done in this area, leading experts to believe that there is a connection between serious head injury and Alzheimer's disease, mostly when head trauma occurs repeatedly. While most of us are not playing football, this is a reminder to always wear your seatbelt when driving or when you are a passenger in a car. Also, remember to wear a helmet when riding a bicycle or motorcycle, or when participating in a sport that recommends or requires one.

This warning to protect our head also goes for navigating treacherous stairs and climbing any kind of ladders. My mom once fell backwards off a ladder while trying to retrieve holiday decorations stored on a high shelf in her garage. She ended up with lots of stitches in the back of her head — and that couldn't have been good for her forthcoming dementia.

As I'm sharing this last recommendation with you, I'm tempted to say, "Fasten your seatbelts, it's going to be a bumpy ride" like Bette Davis's character in *All About Eve*. The truth is, fighting the effects of age can be a bit of a bumpy ride. If being active and challenging ourselves is what we need to do to keep our brain healthy and our cognitive skills intact, then we are going to have to find fun and exciting ways to do that. So if some of those ways pose some risk of injury, we're just going to have to use our brain and take the necessary precautions before we get going.

When I close my eyes and imagine the possibilities for my future, I see myself hiking in one of our beautiful national parks (hopefully with no bears around). I see myself ziplining through a tropical forest (hopefully without encountering mosquitoes). I see myself schussing down a mountain slope (hopefully not bumping into too many moguls) or kayaking down a river (hopefully without rapids). Okay, what if you don't dig this active life that I do and you are thinking, "Joan, I didn't want to zipline when I was in my 30s so why would I fantasize about that for my Third Stage. Well, we all have to come up with our own ideal of this exciting phase of our future. Maybe you see yourself playing chess in an actual tournament or having your own art show. Or auditioning for a Broadway play or swimming with dolphins. Okay, you get the point. It's your life; don't stop living it!

Seriously, if brain researchers have written us the Rx for better brain health and it includes lots of mental and physical activity, then let's follow their orders and get busy having fun. It will certainly help the medicine go down easier.

We're so lucky to live in a time when the findings from such a vast amount of brain research is coming to us at rocket speed. Unlocking the secrets of the brain and having a better understanding of cognitive aging will certainly be one of the biggest challenges of this century as the population of elderly people around the world continues to rise exponentially.

It's up to us, though, to take advantage of all this research, to process the information, to take charge of our health and well-being, and to start thinking like a doctor.

■ ■ ■ ■

PART TWO:
THE BODY

■ ■ ■ ■

"Fall in love with
taking care of your body."
— KIMBERLY SNYDER

CHAPTER 7
WHY CAN'T I LOSE WEIGHT LIKE I LOSE MY KEYS, PHONE, AND SEX DRIVE?

> "I've decided I'll never get down
> to my original weight and I'm
> okay with that. After all,
> 7 pounds 3 oz. is just not realistic."
>
> — UNKNOWN

Do you ever sneak into your bathroom or your closet to quickly change into your PJs so no one sees you naked? Or are you the type to drop your dress and proudly prance around wearing a tiny negligee or less?

It seems to me that no matter which category we fall in, we can still find a reason to obsess over our body. So I thought it would be helpful for all of us to get "naked" and address how our changing body makes us feel, and why it goes through the transitions it does over the decades.

For many, this love/hate relationship begins when we progress from little girls to curvy teens and intensifies when we go away to college and contend with the dreaded *freshman fifteen.* That's when we literally begin to grade our bodies on a scale.

> "There are 3 billion women who don't look like supermodels.
> And only 10 who do."
> — THE BODY SHOP

The next curve likely comes with pregnancy — a deliriously happy time, for sure — though it, too, can leave you with an added fifteen pounds after your bundle of joy has been delivered. Another baby, another fifteen pounds. You can see how this adds up.

This has certainly been the story of my life — my weight has yo-yoed through each and every chapter. After having my first three daughters, I would only change my clothes in the bathroom. There was no prancing around nude for this post-partum body. Not that I was ever the prancing type — or the negligee-wearing type for that matter.

The fact that I spent my mornings perched in front of a camera only added to my body consciousness. I was constantly compared to other women, and inspected for how I looked, how I dressed, and how I was aging. Sure, being on television comes with a ton of perks, but it also comes with a great deal of scrutiny and judgement.

I am just like every other woman out there; sometimes I'm insecure, sometimes I'm aware that I need to take greater control of my health, and sometimes I'm a little like a rudderless ship going around in circles. I tried every promising diet and every fad workout and still, nothing ever worked. I came up with a million reasons why I hadn't lost what I affectionately referred to as my *baby weight.* Those last ten to fifteen pounds can be so hard to shed after each birth. Three daughters, you do the math: $3 \times 15 = 45$ no matter how you fiddle with the numbers. At first it was easy to dismiss the extra pounds as post-pregnancy retention, but years later they were harder to justify.

When the *baby weight* had turned into *toddler weight,* I knew I had to make some serious changes, or I was going to end up carrying it into their teen years! Was it rational to keep blaming my belly on my kids? It sure seemed like it at the time, but that excuse wore thin as time passed.

Of course, we don't have to get pregnant to struggle with weight. This is an issue women wrestle with at all different stages of life.

Throughout much of my career, I was particularly aware of my weight and dress size because I was always being fitted for wardrobe or for a photo shoot. During my 20 years on morning television, I worked with a consultant whose job was to help me buy clothes for the show. Three or four times a year she would take me to New York's fashion district to make selections for the upcoming season. Each time, I cringed when she asked, *"What size are you these days?"* I wanted to tell her, "I'm an eight. Yeah that's right, I'm a svelte, tight, cute, little size eight." But deep down, I also knew that if I bent the truth even a little, clothes would arrive at my dressing room and they wouldn't fit. Even if I fudged and said, "I'm between a 10 and 12," she and I both knew that meant a 12 on a good day.

During our shopping excursions, we spent several days going from showroom to showroom looking at the fashions each clothing manufacturer was selling. Designer showrooms are not like retail stores; there are no racks with an assortment of sizes for us to try on and there are no dressing rooms. Instead, salespeople bring out samples — usually Twiggy-sized ones. By that, I mean size four samples. It was up to me to order the clothes in the size that I *thought* would fit and look good on me.

I never had the chance to try on any of the clothing we ordered until it arrived at the studio several months later. Sometimes I'd put on an outfit that looked absolutely adorable in the showroom size, but it just didn't look the same in a size twelve. Not even close. Ugh!

In addition to a studio wardrobe, we'd always look for at least two or three long gowns for formal events, as I was often invited to state dinners at the White House and to charitable galas. We sometimes had to use our imaginations to predict what else I might need while I was on the road doing stories for GMA. For instance, I never knew when I might have to get down on the floor in exercise gear to demonstrate the latest workout trends, ride a horse in cowboy boots and chaps, or spin around Central Park's Wollman Rink in a cute ice-skating outfit alongside an Olympic champion. Who knew what any given day would bring while hosting a show like GMA? I only knew that I had to be camera-ready at all times!

Once, when the legendary TV program *Hollywood Squares* came to New York City to tape at Radio City Music Hall, I was thrilled to be asked to appear on the show. Joan Rivers was to be the *center square* and around her in the other squares were some other notable New Yorkers including Regis Philbin, Willard Scott from *Today,* Dr. Ruth (the sex therapist), and me.

Unfortunately, what I recall most from that day was arriving for the taping wearing a light pink satin pant suit complete with a long, flowy jacket. I thought it was a glamorous Hollywood look, but as I made my way to the stage, a greeter from the show ran up to me and said, "Hi, Miss Lunden, oh, you look beautiful. I didn't know you were expecting."

Ouch!

I *wasn't* expecting.

In my defense I had delivered my third daughter, Sarah, six months earlier, but I certainly didn't think I looked as if I were still carrying her! Apparently that young man didn't know the golden rule: never ask a woman if she is pregnant! I was so embarrassed.

I had to shake it off and try not to appear ruffled, even though I was. It was a moment I've never forgotten.

As I approached my 39th birthday, everything began to crystalize for me. I had seen a magazine cover featuring Farrah Fawcett, Jaclyn Smith, and Kate Jackson — the three gorgeous ladies starring on *Charlie's Angels.*

The headline read: *Fit, Forty, and Fabulous.* YES! I wanted to be *that.* I had one year to make it happen. *Could I pull it off?* All I knew was that I desperately wanted to.

But time passed by and like always, life got in the way. (Read that as I was busy at work, busy as a mom, and busy dealing with the daily struggles that so many women experience.) Then about a month later, I had what I can only describe as a real *aha* moment. It came when I was interviewing a representative from the American Heart Association who had brought a quiz for our GMA viewers to help them assess their risk for cardiovascular disease and heart attack. As the interview progressed, I realized I was failing the test miserably.

Inactive? Check.

Making bad food choices? Check.

Stressed out? Overweight? Not getting enough sleep? Check, check, and check.

When I realized what this meant, I nearly had a panic attack live on the air.

I was almost 40! I knew I was putting off important medical tests because I was afraid of the results, and if I'm going to be completely honest, I simply didn't want to go to the doctor because I didn't want to get on the scale.

I also knew that my marriage was ending,

and that meant I'd eventually be back out there "on the market" again. If I wanted to have a shot at rebooting my life, I needed to get my booty in shape.

After endless attempts at dieting and camouflage dressing, followed by more than my share of pizza and French fries (did I really just confess that?!), I sought the guidance of some really encouraging experts.

With their help, I dramatically changed the way I approached eating. I aligned my mind, body, and spirit. It's amazing what we can accomplish when we are motivated, inspired, or just plain scared of the consequences inactive choices bring. I lost almost fifty pounds, learned to eat healthily, and added physical exercise and more play into my life.

I openly shared that journey in *Joan Lunden's Healthy Cooking* because I knew I wasn't the only one seeking a better way to live. I was so excited about my newly energized, svelte, fit, effervescent self that I couldn't wait to divulge all that I had learned to my viewers and readers.

My physical transformation gave me a new vitality and propelled me to keep going until I was back to my old — or I should say *former* — energetic self.

Feeling fit again changed how I presented

myself, how I walked into a room. It affected how I thought about my potential, and it even influenced the kind of vacation I took. Now I was choosing tall mountains to climb and white sandy beaches where I could wear my newly purchased bikini! That's right, I said *bikini,* not one piece and *not* tankini! Watch out Angels . . . I was back!

It absolutely changed the course of my life. I ended up meeting my husband, Jeff! I firmly believe that it was my newfound confidence and zest for living that brought us together. Jeff was ten years my junior, yet our relationship seemed so natural and comfortable. That didn't just happen. I made it happen by taking control of my health and fitness.

By the way, there was a ten-year age difference in *both* of my marriages. When I married my first husband, I was 29 years old and he was 39. Then twenty years later, when I was 49, I remarried, and again he was 39. Oh yeah, I can attest to the fact that marrying a younger man is one of the great secrets to feeling, looking, and staying younger than my years!

By the time the big 5-0 was just around the corner, I felt so vibrant that I didn't even question having children again, two sets of twins no less. So as you can imagine my 50s were not the typical 50s. Instead of planning my retirement, I was chasing babies all over the place, and I loved every minute of it.

Meanwhile, while I may have been living the life of a new mom, there's no getting around it that my body was in its 50s and had already started going through the natural changes women experience through the decades. With those changes came muscle loss and a slower metabolism, to say nothing of droopy body parts. According to the American College of Sports Medicine, we lose an average of 3 to 5 percent of our muscle mass each decade after the age of 35 if we don't do anything about it. This means that our resting metabolic rate declines an average of 2 to 3 percent every decade. But once we are in our 50s the aging process puts the pedal to the metal.

Holy S&@! I felt like I was Chicken Little. "My metabolism is falling, my metabolism is falling!" And we all know what that means . . . . it means we can be eating the exact amount we did at 40 — not a morsel more — and still gain weight. It also means shedding those pounds is a lot harder.

We may suddenly find that the same weight-loss methods that worked for us prior to menopause just don't work like they used to. This is because of the relationship between our estrogen and our insulin levels. Insulin is a fat storage hormone, and estrogen is what sensitizes our body to insulin. When our estrogen levels are optimal, we don't need as much insulin, but as we age and enter menopause, our estrogen levels decline. That's when we become vulnerable to the effects of our insulin. As our insulin levels rise, our body starts storing more fat, especially around our midsection.

Once we're staring down 60, it becomes insanely easy to let ten or twenty pounds sneak onto our body without realizing it. Okay, at least without *admitting* it. We all know when we've gained weight. But if you're like me, we also delude ourselves into thinking we can lose it just as easily. Maybe shedding 3 to 5 pounds was easier before menopause. Maybe you remember thinking, "Oh, it's only 5 pounds!" A bag of sugar is 5 pounds! Maybe that was true before menopause, but certainly not afterward. Our entire body morphs into a new shape. Suddenly our clothes don't seem to fit us like they used to. I almost cried when I found that my favorite jeans were cutting into my waistline and (*gasp*), leaving a mark! Goodbye bikini!

So let's talk about how our bodies are changing and what we can do about that unwanted excess weight. If we better understand what is naturally occurring during the aging process, we can all improve what needs to be improved and accept the rest.

The human body is made up of bones, water, fat, and lean tissue (i.e., muscles and organs). While researching for this book, I was shocked to learn that after age 20, our daily energy expenditure (the calories we burn daily) decreases by about 150 calories each decade. This is due to the fact that our body is losing muscle mass and gaining fat. According to the American Council on Exercise, that decrease continues and becomes most dramatic for women when we hit age 50. That means if we easily burned 2,000 calories a day when we were an energetic 20-year-old, we may only be burning about 1,550 calories a day when we are in our 50s.

But here's the good news: We used to think all of the changes that came with aging were determined by our genes. Now research shows that only 30 percent of health and longevity is controlled by genetics and that 70 percent is in our hands to control. That's right, our genes play a far less important role than lifestyle choices, diet, and health maintenance.

"Your body is a reflection of your lifestyle."
— UNKNOWN

More recent research conducted by Calico Life Sciences and published in the *Journal of Genetics* went as far as saying that genetics only account for 7 percent of longevity. Their studies show that people's life spans are much more likely to be similar to their spouse's than to their sibling's since they tend to live the same lifestyle. Researchers also report that non-genetic factors, such as having access to healthy food and clean water, have the strongest influence over our longevity, as do avoiding habits such as smoking.

Some of these changes are inevitable of course, but our lifestyle choices may slow or speed up the process.

We talked before about losing muscle as we age. This muscle loss has a name — it is known as *sarcopenia,* and it's not only one of the major causes of weight gain, it can also contribute to weakness as we get older. In addition to thinning bones, it can lead to falls and broken hips. So no, it wasn't necessarily that last glass of wine that made you a bit unbalanced; just blame it on sarcopenia.

123

She's a bi@#h!

The only way to combat the loss of muscle is to make sure that we have some physical activity in our life. Strength training is especially effective at rebuilding muscle mass. And while we're at it, we should also do some cardio and limit our caloric intake. Sorry, I had to say it.

I read somewhere that as a person ages, their appetite begins to wane . . . Well, there it is! Proof that I am *not* aging!

I know this all means that I not only have to eat smarter, I must also figure out how to get enough exercise to rebuild and maintain the muscle that I've lost. I do my best to get both cardio and strength training into my schedule. Some weeks I'm better at that than others, but I'm not perfect. The last time I looked, I wasn't Jane Fonda. By the way, have you seen her lately? She looks *amazing* and she's in her 80s! That should be an inspiration to us all.

I feel so much better after my workouts, but admittedly it's not always easy motivating myself to do them. I wonder if I could get Jane to call me each morning to roust me out of bed and into the gym. There's a business idea in that. I'd sign up for a daily automated message from her, saying, "Hi, it's Jane Fonda and I'm calling to remind you to get your butt moving and do your workout, so when you reach 80 your body can look like mine!" Wouldn't you?

For a lot of people, the hardest part of getting into and sticking with a good exercise routine is taking that step and actually doing something about it. Sometimes all it takes is a little help from our friends.

Quite a while ago I got some of that friendly help and its impact has stayed with me to this day. I was in Atlanta, Georgia, covering one of the national Democratic conventions for *Good Morning America.* The GMA staff of producers and writers were checking in to their rooms at the Omni Hotel. As the huge glass elevator made its way up to our floor, my colleagues were making dates to go out for dinner or to meet in the gym. As I listened to their enthusiastic plans, I felt a whoosh of shame come over me. I knew I needed to start exercising, but all I'd done so far was beat myself up over it — and by the way, that never burns calories.

Suddenly I heard myself say, "Oh my gosh, I can't believe it, I forgot to bring my sneakers." Our weatherman, Spencer Christian, was on that elevator with me. He had heard me talk about wanting to start exercising for so many years that he just couldn't keep silent any longer. He said, "You're always complaining about needing to lose weight, Joan. Stop talking about it, and just do it. Get a pair of sneakers or come barefoot but meet me at the gym."

Really, Spencer? Really? How brave of him! I let him live because I knew he was absolutely right.

Whether he meant to or not, Spencer totally called me out in that crowded elevator. He went one step further and challenged me to join him. I accepted the challenge, borrowed a pair of sneakers, and later that evening, found him at the gym doing sit-ups and lifting weights. He had always been super trim and fit.

When I looked around, I didn't know where to begin; that gym might as well have been an alien spaceship. The equipment seemed so foreign to me, but I'd ridden a bicycle as a child, so I got on a stationary one and began pedaling. A few minutes felt like hours, so I slowed down. I felt like a gerbil spinning on its wheel but getting nowhere. Spencer looked up from his weights and asked, "What's going on, Lunden?" I had to tell him that I hated it. I felt like I was pedaling to a place I did *not* want to go.

He tried not to be frustrated with me, but

126

I could tell he was. He said, "Look, it just means that you need to try something else in this gym. You don't give in; you just keep trying different forms of exercise until you find something that works for you. You don't have to love it, but you need to enjoy it enough to stick with it. If you hate it, you'll *never* stick with it."

For the duration of the convention, Spencer made gym dates with me as a way to keep me motivated. He called them *non-negotiable, unbreakable gym dates.* His aim was to help me form a habit of working out.

Sometime later, Spencer pulled me aside and said, "I hope your time in the gym was the kick in the ass that you needed. Now it's up to you to keep it up." I'm not going to tell you that I love going to the gym. Some days are better than others. But I go, I always try to do my best, and I remain thankful to Spencer for motivating me.

We all discover our own path to the fitness regimen that works for us. It doesn't mean that we need to become gym rats or take up CrossFit (I mean, unless you want to), but it does mean that we should have some regular physical activity in our lives. If you look at countries where people live longer, such as Greece, Italy, and Japan, you will note that the population there generally enjoys a nutritious diet and leads a more physically active, less stressful life.

As we age, it becomes more difficult for us to recover after taking a tumble. I've unfortunately taken a few awkward falls myself in the past few years, and it seems as if it took forever to heal. Shooting video of my four younger kids while skiing down a steep mountain seemed like a good idea at the time. That is until the tips of my skis crossed, and I ended up with a face full of snow, a small fracture in my left fibula, and some really awkward footage of me going downhill. When that injury finally healed, a few too many hours playing tennis led to another fracture, this time to my left foot. It took eight months to mend. My days of wearing high heels seem to be over, but maybe that's not such a bad thing after all.

My propensity for breaks could be due to my density — *bone density* that is. In addition to muscle loss, lower levels of estrogen during menopause can cause women to lose some matter in their bones. Low bone density is actually quite common, affecting as many as 54 million Americans. According to the National Osteoporosis Foundation, women are four times more likely than men to develop osteoporosis. In fact, one out of every two women over the age of 50 is likely to break a bone due to this condition. Well, I've done my part for driving up that average.

We women were originally engineered to have babies in our teens and 20s, so our reproductive hormone levels naturally start dropping in our 30s. As our estrogen levels fall, we can expect the onset of perimenopause, which usually begins in our 40s, but can start as early as our 30s or even sooner. During this time, estrogen levels become quite erratic and progesterone levels also decline. We begin to experience irregular periods and symptoms such as hot flashes, sleeplessness, night sweats, mood changes, fatigue, and weight gain. And still it can be years before our last menstrual period.

Menopause is defined as when we have experienced 12 consecutive months without a period. The average age for the onset of menopause is 51. It marks the end of our reproductive years and the time when our ovaries stop making estrogen.

Menopause can cause a lot more than annoying hot flashes that bring us to a slow boil. It can make some women feel as if they're in a constant state of PMS. You know the symptoms: You're moody, sad, irritable, and lethargic. Supposedly, hot flashes last about two years, but for 15 to

20 percent of women, they never go away. Just thinking about it raises my temperature. Is it just me or is it hot in here?

To be totally frank, men *really* don't understand just how horrible these hot flashes can be. A friend of mine bought a new car. After a week or so, she noticed the air conditioning didn't work. She said it was blowing warm air. Every time she brought it into the auto shop for service, the manager dismissed her complaint. It was on her sixth visit to get the car fixed that he finally said, "My wife has the same problem. She's always hot in the car, even when I blast the air. You know, you are both women of a certain age."

Oh no. Did he really say that?

He did.

When it comes to hot flashes, they can arrive suddenly, flooding the body with intense heat, causing mostly our faces, necks, and chests to flush. They can also cause intense sweating and your heart to beat faster. If we lose too much body heat, we can feel chilled afterward. One minute you want to throw all the covers off and the next you're freezing cold. It's believed that as estrogen levels drop, the hypothalamus — that part of the brain that regulates our body temperature — gets so overactive, it sends a chemical alert to the rest of our body telling it that we're overheating. The body then releases the heat, and a cold flash follows. I have found that having one leg outside of the covers and one under makes for a pretty good compromise. Who is with me on this theory? Sticking your head in the freezer is also a great quick fix.

Hot flashes last about one to five minutes (or an eternity if you are the one enduring them!). They may occur a few times a week for some women and daily for others. Are we having fun yet? When hot flashes are really severe, they may strike 4 or 5 times an hour or 20 to 30 times a day. Yikes! Apparently, alcohol, caffeine, spicy foods, and smoking can all intensify hot flashes and night sweats. Note which of these can be a trigger for you and make every effort to avoid them. Drinking hot liquids and dressing too warmly are culprits for a lot of women as well. Realizing that cashmere can be at fault has saved me a lot of money!

Fun Fact: Some men also experience hormonal changes. This period of change for them is officially called *andropause,* aka *manopause.* About 20 percent of men over 60 experience it because of a decrease in their testosterone production, although it can come on sooner for some men. I have a friend who was in his 30s when he entered premature andropause. It was very scary for him because at the time, he was a personal trainer, unable to figure out why he was gaining weight and losing stamina. When he went to see his doctor, his physician said, "You've got the testosterone levels of an 80-year-old man." Something needed to change and fast. Once he recognized the symptoms, including lowered energy levels, depression, decreased muscle strength, and decreased sex drive, he was able to manage it. Wait, I didn't hear any mention of hot flashes. While I wouldn't wish them on anyone, how did only women get stuck with those?!

While hot flashes are completely annoying, there is one other thing about menopause that is even more frustrating — the redistribution of body fat from our hips to our abdomen. What I'm talking about here is *belly fat!* Again, the normal decreased level of estrogen at this stage of life is what's responsible for the migration of stored body fat from our hips and thighs to our midriff. We carry fat on our hips and thighs during our childbearing years to help offset the weight of a growing belly. When that is no longer necessary, it begins its journey to the belly. While pregnant belly fat is a necessary evil, during menopause it's just plain evil!

I always had a great waistline. If you are like me, then I know you find this shift in body weight simply maddening too.

I've not only been researching why this happens to women, but what potential dangers it presents and what we can do about it. We've already talked about the delicate balance between estrogen and insulin and how it can make it difficult to lose weight. But when this age-related change in estrogen occurs, it can also make women insulin resistant, which brings with it an increased risk of metabolic syndrome, Type 2 diabetes, and heart disease. I don't want to sound like a broken record, but the best course of action is exercise and eating healthily. All too often, however, women will try to combat their expanding waistline with a very-low-calorie diet, which, believe it or not, is the *worst* thing you can do since research has shown that restricting calories causes even greater loss of muscle mass and a decline in metabolic rate. While you may see short-term results, the long-term effect may be quite different. I tried that tactic unsuccessfully, and the weight not only re-appeared, but I was left feeling lethargic.

As we age, our maximum heart rate — that's the fastest speed our heart is able to go — also begins to decrease. This slowing down of the heart may play a role in our waning capacity for aerobic exercise. When I'm at the gym these days, trying to push myself as hard as I can, I'm increasingly aware that it's not the same as when I was younger. Recently, I've made a conscious effort to look for fitness classes that will push me and keep my heart rate up, but still be more realistically my speed.

But none of the changes I've addressed so far likely catch us by surprise more than the changes that occur in our sexual desire and in our sex life itself. A loss of libido or decreased sex drive is quite common, although it is different for every woman. Some barely notice it, while others never recover it. Other women will experience what anthropologist Margaret Mead called PMZ — post menopausal zest — not to be confused with *TMZ,* the celebrity gossip television show.

Sex after menopause is probably one of the least discussed aspects of this stage of life. We shouldn't freak out over the loss of sexual desire because many women will be able to regain it. We may not necessarily enjoy the same level of sexual drive we had in our 30s and 40s, but we can, indeed, get some of our mojo back. In researching what to do to kick-start this loss of desire, I found one sex therapist who recommended showing up in the bedroom once a week naked with only a smile on your face. I'm trying to imagine that scene in my bedroom right now, and candidly I'm chuckling . . . not sure what my husband's reaction would be.

For some, it's not only a matter of desire, it's a matter of physical discomfort or distress during intercourse. Sex can be *painful* for many women after menopause. In fact, according to the National Menopause Foundation, between 17 to 45 percent of women will experience discomfort ranging from a tight feeling to severe pain. The condition is known as the genitourinary syndrome of menopause or GSM, and it is due to decreasing estrogen levels as well as a decline in other sex steroid hormones. These shifts in our hormone levels cause the vaginal tissue to become thin and dry, which, in turn, can cause friction, irritation, burning, and pain during sex. Many women also experience frequent nighttime urination or pain with urination. Some women describe the pain they have while having sex as feeling like sandpaper.

There are safe and effective treatments for this condition, but studies show a large percentage of women wait a long time to seek treatment, and some don't get any at all. According to Dr. JoAnn Pinkerton, executive director of the North American Menopause Society and professor of obstetrics and gynecology at the University of Virginia Health System, "Painful sex is highly prevalent in older women and negatively affects sexual intimacy and quality of life, but women are embarrassed to talk about it." One woman I know actually said to her husband, "Can't we just be good friends?"

When women experience these changes in desire and sexual enjoyment, they often avoid sex, and that frequently leads to worry about how their husbands will react. It can be difficult for couples since a withdrawal from physical intimacy can create feelings of rejection for our mate. In most cases, it isn't rejection so much as a fear of pain or discomfort. Well, in some cases, it may be rejection. I'll leave that one up to you.

My suggestion: live, laugh, and lube.

If you are experiencing mild vaginal irritation or discomfort, the North American Menopause Society says the first thing to do is to stop using any kind of soap on the inner parts of your vulva. They also recommend using only unscented toilet paper, washing your underwear in detergents free of dyes and perfumes, and ceasing the use of fabric softeners and anti-cling laundry products. Finally, they suggest avoiding any lotions and perfumed products on the inner vulva.

There are a number of different topical vaginal treatments to help relieve pain during intercourse. If you have mild to moderate vaginal dryness, you can start by looking for simple, over-the-counter (OTC), non-prescription vaginal moisturizers and lubricants at your local drugstore. These come in liquid or gel form and work by reducing the friction associated with dry genital tissue. They can also be found on Amazon if you feel too embarrassed to be in public for fear you may bump into your mother-in-law at CVS.

If you have more severe pain and the OTC lubricants don't work for you, your doctor can prescribe a low-dose vaginal estrogen product that comes in either cream, suppository, or ring form. All are intended to be minimally absorbed (unlike hormone replacement therapy, which enters the bloodstream) to restore thickness and flexibility to vaginal tissues.

Lubricants work well for many women, although I have a friend who said she tried every type on the market until she got so tired of playing bedroom slip and slide, she had to look for other solutions.

She turned to a treatment called the Mona-Lisa Touch. It is a minimally invasive treatment for vaginal atrophy done in a doctor's office. A CO_2 laser is used to deliver energy to the vaginal tissue. It is similar to laser facial treatments in that the laser makes micro-abrasions, or tiny scratches, in the vaginal wall, which stimulate the growth of new blood vessels. The treatment is reported by the manufacturer to be nearly painless, takes about five minutes, and requires no anesthesia. It does require several sessions and a *booster* session every 18 months or so. It was approved by the FDA in 2004; however, most insurance companies won't cover the cost, which averages $2,400.

After menopause the vaginal tissue can not only be drier, it can also lose its elasticity so that the vagina becomes narrower and shorter. (This can also occur in women of any age who have had cancer treatments or surgery to lower their risk of cancer.) Women suffering with this issue can turn to vaginal dilator therapy. A vaginal dilator is a tube-shaped device that is used to stretch the vagina. Kits are available, which include different sized dilators, from small to large. The length of treatment varies from woman to woman.

While 1 in 3 women are said to experience these issues, many women have no real idea of what they should expect with menopause. The problem is that despite living in a world where people seem to openly talk about practically everything, we're still relatively mum on the subjects of menopause and mojo.

Adding to the problem are doctors who don't always recognize the symptoms as being related to decreasing hormone levels. In such cases, they may prescribe sleep medications for a woman experiencing disrupted sleep and tranquilizers for relief of the anxiety associated with lack of sleep. If we stop numbing women, and just talk more about this stuff, we'd realize how normal it all is and we'd collectively find more effective solutions.

Our aging bodies are going to present us with new challenges that can be annoying, embarrassing, uncomfortable, inconvenient, and even painful. However, I believe that having a better understanding of how our body works and anticipating what the changes are likely to be, can help us all feel better about our bodies and remind us that we are not alone in this evolving life experience.

If these problems are familiar to you, don't

just suffer in silence — seek help. By opening up this dialogue, I hope to help us all feel less isolated and scared. I want us to be empowered and to draw strength from one another. I certainly learned a lot in writing this book and I hope that reading it is helping you too.

Finally, this chapter is a friendly reminder that we should keep going to our gynecologist even after menopause. Self-care is vital at every age.

CHAPTER 8
STRONG IS THE NEW SKINNY

"Be the kind of woman that when your feet hit the floor each morning the devil says, 'Oh crap, she's up.' "

— UNKNOWN

If you had asked me when I was in my 30s what I wanted to change about my body, I would have said without a doubt, "I want to be skinny!" Today, while I watch my weight, the answer to that same question would be different. I'd say, "I want to be strong, healthy, and resilient!" After a recent workout, I found myself standing in my bathroom deciding whether or not to step on the scale. I don't know about you, but I even take off my earrings before I weigh myself. On this day, however, I stood there looking at my naked image in the mirror and consciously decided that the number on the scale was not what I needed to see. Instead I opted to just look at the strong confident healthy image staring back at me. I asked myself whether I felt energetic, happy, or stressed? It occurred to me in that moment that I had come to a turning point in my life. I was now measuring my fitness by how I was dealing with life — by how I was managing my health. That was when I realized I cared more about being strong than about being skinny.

How would *you* describe a strong woman? I'm guessing you wouldn't say it's someone who can bench press more than their trainer. In fact, I imagine you're more likely to say she's a someone who has the fortitude and the resilience to elegantly navigate the challenging times in her life and who shows strength in her ability to lift others up when they need help. Someone who honors her own and others' health.

Interestingly, women tend to experience more stress, more chronic diseases, and more anxiety and depression than men. Women are also more likely to be victims of violence, and in some countries, women still don't have the same human rights as men. However, despite all of the social inequality that women have experienced throughout history, we have always lived longer than men.

So with that little tidbit, I think it's totally

fair to add *longevity* to our definition of a strong woman.

Of course, that fact has left the scientific community asking the age-old question, why *do* women live longer than men?

There are a number of different thoughts on why we are able to survive life's harshest conditions and live the longest.

A study out of the Southern University of Denmark compared data from seven of the worst times in history — times when a population was exposed to such extreme conditions as famines, epidemics, and enslavement — and found women were able to survive for much longer periods of time than men, no matter what their age. The study also found that newborn girls were able to survive extreme mortality hazards better than the newborn boys. Research suggests that hormonal differences may explain this gender mortality gap. For example, estrogens, which are found in larger quantities in women, tend to have an anti-inflammatory effect, whereas testosterone, found in larger amounts in men, may actually suppress the immune systems. Maybe this explains why men deal with the common cold — or should I say, a "man cold" — the way that they do!, or why they can't get pregnant. Nature knows a man

143

would be unbearable pregnant!

At Michigan State University biologists are studying differences in our cells, specifically our *mast cells,* a type of white blood cell that is part of the immune system. Women's mast cells make and store more inflammatory substances, such as histamine and serotonin, which are actually responsible for many mast cells-associated diseases including IBS, migraine headaches, airway congestion, and shortness of breath.

When the mast cells are activated by stress or allergens, they release those inflammatory substances, which can then activate a more aggressive immune response in women than men typically exhibit. Men are less prone to have hyperactive immune disorders. While this hardly sounds like an advantage, there is another side to this story: These mast cells are the very first immune cells to become activated in response to an infection. They are critical not only in fighting viruses and bacteria, but in developing a protective immunity to prevent future infections. If you're still unclear why women's immune systems are superior, I have one word for you: moms.

Another factor in women's longevity is our tendency to develop cardiovascular disease about ten years later in life than men. We usually develop it in our 70s and 80s, whereas men develop it in their 50s and 60s. There are several theories as to why this is the case. Estrogen offers us some protection from heart disease, until, of course, we finish menopause and our estrogen levels drop. Researchers also believe that estrogen has a positive effect on the inner layer of the artery wall, which helps keep our blood vessels flexible. And finally, there is research from Stanford University Medical School that found that women's bodies are better at dealing with insensitivity to insulin, which controls our blood sugar. The researchers who studied people with this insensitivity found that women were less likely than men to have high blood pressure and high triglycerides — both of which are known to increase the risk of heart disease.

That being said, heart disease is still the leading cause of death in women, mainly because women are either misdiagnosed or don't seek treatment when they have symptoms of a heart attack. The larger percentage of women now being treated for high blood pressure and cholesterol also indicates that we need better and earlier screening, so please ladies, be vigilant about taking care of your heart!

Another theory about women's superior

longevity has to do with iron. We all need iron to make hemoglobin. However, as one of the few minerals we can't eliminate (except through blood loss), iron's accumulation in the body can be problematic. When it rises to toxic levels, it can increase the risks of cancer and heart disease. Because women may be more iron deficient during our reproductive years compared to men, we don't have to contend with the concern of toxic iron levels, at least not until later in life.

Women also have the advantage of having two X chromosomes. By contrast, men have one X and one Y. A woman's second X chromosome may act as a backup should any of the genes on the other X be damaged. That's women for you. We're always prepared with extra supplies: lipstick, snacks, tissues, and extra X chromosomes just in case we need backup. We are, quite literally, ready for anything even on a genetic level!

Finally, women may also have a basic biological advantage because the female role in reproduction is vital to survival — we give birth, we nurse our babies, and care for them during their early years . . . okay, during all of their years. Let's just say that men's role in reproduction is limited, and for that reason, longevity in men may not be as vital to the continuation of the species.

While we can't necessarily bench press what men can, this all makes for a pretty compelling case that women are the stronger sex in that we have a stronger purpose for living. Now, before we get all full of ourselves, having these *natural* advantages doesn't necessarily guarantee longevity when poor lifestyle choices such as obesity, alcohol use, and smoking are factored in. We're not really in the clear, ladies.

According to one study by the Center for Retirement Research at Boston College, even though lifespans have increased in the U.S. over the decades, life expectancy for women in this country has stalled, and in some rural areas of the U.S. it has actually been falling.

While there has been a large life expectancy gap between men and women in the past, some researchers predict it could even up by 2030. Wait! We can't let this happen. We are the stronger sex! Remember? Nature needs us!

So what is causing this? There are a number of reasons that have contributed to this downward trend in women's lifespan. Obesity is, of course, right up there at the top of the list. More recently it has become a notable trend in younger women who have had a difficult time shedding pounds after pregnancy. That statistic breaks my heart since I can relate to how difficult it is to rid oneself of that weight.

Women also have to deal with an overwhelming amount of stress in today's world, especially as they try to balance their work and family responsibilities. This stress can carry significant risk later in life. Just think about how much has changed for all of us in America since the time of our mothers and grandmothers. Our lives feel far more overwhelming and chaotic than ever before as we strive to *do it all*.

Sadly, there's also been an overall increase in suicides, prescription drug abuse, and alcohol-related deaths, which have played a role in our declining longevity. And it doesn't help that in rural areas, there is less access to quality medical care.

One of the facts I find particularly difficult to understand is how smoking, with all of the public information available about the dangers it poses, is yet another major contributor to the trend toward earlier morbidity among women. Lung cancer is the leading cancer killer among women in the U.S., taking the lives of more women each year than breast, ovarian, and uterine cancers combined. The fact that there has been a decline in smoking by men and an increase in smoking rates among women contributes to turning the tide in longevity rates.

So where does this leave us?

Women have fought for decades to be equal to men. Since the birth of the Women's Movement five decades ago, we are better educated than ever before, many have more fulfilling and better paying jobs, and most of us are having fewer children. I know, with seven kids, I really screw up that average. However, this lifestyle also means that many of us have less free time, more stress, less sex, more divorce, and all too often compromised health. When we say "equality," we don't mean in mortality rates, do we?

> "If evolution really works, how come mothers only have two hands?"
> — MILTON BERLE

The reality is that women today have a lot more on their plate. We make up just under 50 percent of our full-time workforce and in many families, women are bringing in at least half the household income. What all this translates to is that many of us are working *two* full-time jobs — the job we have outside the home and that full-time job waiting for us back at home taking care of the house, raising children, grocery shopping, cooking dinner, doing laundry, helping with homework, and sometimes also taking care of elderly parents. It's enough to make anyone exhausted, not to mention cranky.

But we're pulling it off, right? We have it all and we're doing it all?

But at what cost?

When our lifestyle is overwhelming, it influences our sleep patterns, our energy, our stress levels — and all this can have an impact on our weight, health, longevity, *and* happiness.

I thought we were striving to be strong!

I know I used to look at young supermodels and envy them, but now it's a strong woman of any age, fit and full of enthusiasm, with a glow to her skin and a sparkle in her eyes, who impresses and inspires me. And hey, if that woman also happens to have muscular, well-toned arms, I'm in total awe of her. I know that she is a woman who honors her body, who invests in her health, and takes time to relax and recharge. You've probably heard the saying, *You can't pour from an empty cup; you must take care of yourself first,* and it is so true. To be the best mom, the best wife, or the best friend possible, we must first be a best friend to ourselves.

Let's all make *strong* the new *skinny.*

CHAPTER 9
BECOME THE CEO
OF YOUR HEALTH

"We have to care about our bodies
and what we put in them. Women
have to take the time to focus on our
mental health — take time for self,
for the spiritual, without feeling guilty
or selfish. The world will see you the
way you see you and treat you the
way you treat yourself."

— BEYONCÉ

Your body is just that — *yours.* You are the
only one listening to it, monitoring it daily.
The only way you can protect it is to take
responsibility for it. How do you do this?

Imagine if we treated our bodies with the
same respect we treat our cars.

I happen to love this analogy, so stick with
me.

If you're driving down the road and the
little orange idiot light comes on reminding
you that service is required, you take your

car in to find out what's wrong with it, right? Because, of course, you want your car to keep running in good condition for as long as possible, right?

Well then, why don't we use that same level of care with our bodies?

How many of us have had aches and pains — the equivalent of *little orange idiot lights* — that we've ignored as if they'll fix themselves? How many of us are on schedule for our annual physicals? Who among us has visited their dermatologist for an annual skin check? Who has seen their gynecologist recently? Ask those questions at your next *girls' lunch,* and I bet most of you will have your tail between your legs. *Why don't you* make *those appointments?* Too busy? Need to find a new doctor? Maybe you don't want to hear any bad news, be told you need to drop a bad habit — or worse, that you have to lose weight? Oh no, thanks, I'm good! Maybe I'll wait till next year! Well *that,* ladies, is the wrong choice, and I am here to be that annoying friend who prods you to change your ways — to make and keep those appointments! Yes, I am because I don't want you to break down in the middle of life's freeway during rush hour traffic.

Many women view taking time for themselves, that is, tending to their physical and emotional wellness, as being selfish. But it's really the opposite. Taking care of our health is the greatest gift we can give those we love. We need to commit to taking care of our body right now. Just like when they tell us on the planes to put the oxygen mask on ourselves first before we try to help anyone else. I know I jumped metaphors, but I think I'm making my point here.

If you're anything like me, going to that doctor's appointment can sometimes feel like going to the principal's office. Do you worry that you might get scolded? "Oh Ms. Lunden, you weigh eight pounds more than your last physical." Or does your mind run away with you? *Should I just be honest and confess that I fell off the exercise wagon? I'll shape up and get back with the program; I swear I will. Will she call me out for being lazy? Maybe I should also tell her that I'm having trouble sleeping at night, waking up two or three times with hot flashes that leave me wiped out the next day. Uh oh, I just remembered that I didn't shave my legs, and this gown is pretty short. Will she notice?*

Just the experience of being in a doctor's office can be uncomfortable and intimidating for some people. You know the drill. You're told to change out of your warm comfortable clothes into that flimsy paper gown! Why aren't those ties ever long enough? Do you think the people who designed those things have a chuckle knowing that our butt will be hanging out?

So now you're wearing a disposable gown that crinkles when you move and requires you to gingerly maneuver yourself onto a cold table covered in that thin white paper that sticks to your exposed thighs

Warning: those gowns rip really easy. Take it from me, I tried pulling one out from under me and when the doctor came back in the room, I had half the gown crumpled in my hand rather than being on my naked body.

Oh, and look, isn't this fun, my legs are dangling off the end of the table like I'm ten years old again. Yep, now I feel like I'm at the top of my game, ready to talk with the doctor about the details of my health. Vulnerable? You bet. Nervous? Of course. Top of my game? Hardly. Hello, did you just hear me say I'm half naked, in a cold room, sitting on a piece of paper?

Newsflash: We are *not* at the top of our game in that outfit.

So now the doctor asks how we've been doing, and if we have been taking care of ourselves? With a completely straight face, some of us will say we are living an amazingly healthy life, exercising regularly, and eating healthily too. And maybe we are doing all of those things. But then again, maybe some of us might be stretching the truth just a little bit. C'mon. We've all done this. But why? Why do we do this with the very person who is there to help us? I think we simply don't want to look bad. But not unlike a defense attorney, they can't help us if we don't tell them everything.

Women avoid going to a doctor for a lot of these reasons. Either we're completely sticking our heads in the sand about potential ailments, or, as I've already admitted, we don't want to step on a scale.

Don't laugh — you know it's true! Maybe if they just let us "adjust" their scale a bit before they weigh us.

I'll even admit to this one. I've pushed back appointments with my internist so I could have more time to lose weight. Can you believe it? What is this — a first date? Honestly, my wedding day was less stressful than this. I don't know why I feel this way! But I do, and I know I am not alone.

We all know how the story ends when we push something off this way. It never really happens. And sometimes that actually makes things worse.

Of course, as I tell you this, I am reminded

of the time that we did *Good Morning America* live for two weeks from Australia and New Zealand.

When we landed in Queenstown and made our way from the airport to the hotel, Charlie Gibson and I saw several storefronts advertising bungee jumping. New Zealand is where bungee jumping started, so I looked to Charlie and said, "You know what they say; when in Rome . . . Let's find that famous bungee jumping bridge and have a go at it."

The network executives would never have allowed us to do it, so we made a plan to sneak out of the hotel early the next morning with a camera crew.

When we arrived at the bungee bridge, we paid our $75 and signed all of the required liability waivers. We were then instructed to step on a scale and stick out our hand. They were going to write our weight on our hand with a magic marker so the bridge operators could calibrate the length of bungee cord needed.

Wait. What? Step on a scale?

"Oh no," I said, "I'll jump off that rusty 17-story bridge hovering dangerously over a narrow river gorge, but no way am I stepping on that scale!"

Can you imagine?

Every female backed away from the scale.

Only when we discovered that the weight would be measured in kilos and confirmed that none of us knew how to convert kilos into pounds, did we all agree to proceed.

Telling this story always makes me chuckle; however, it's not funny when our weight prevents us from going to the doctor for potentially life-saving tests. There can be very dangerous consequences to putting off that gynecological exam, mammogram, colonoscopy, or the bare-naked head-to-toe skin check.

Knowledge holds power when it comes to staying in charge of our health and keeping ahead of disease. Avoiding doctors because we fear bad news really can be deadly.

We are all bombarded with scary health information these days. It can make us feel doomed in advance. One study by the British research group Health2020 found that one-third of people who consciously put off seeing their doctor do so because they fear hearing bad news. The report said that these people are more comfortable gambling with their health than facing their concerns head on. Of course, the problem with that approach is that early intervention is critical for many conditions such as cancer. Not seeing a doctor can allow a condition to worsen. In the case of cancer, finding it early can mean a good prognosis, whereas finding it at a late stage can sometimes mean it's incurable. For some people, though, the fear of bad news can be so overwhelming, it eclipses common sense.

But imagine the alternative: hearing bad news when it might be too late. *Time* is our friend when it comes to protecting our health. Knowing about it sooner is better than discovering it later. I'm incredibly thankful that I went for my yearly screenings so that I found my breast cancer at an early enough stage. I was able to be treated and now here I am sharing that good news with you. Early detection can save your life. I believe it saved mine.

Self-Care Is Never Selfish

Okay, so here I am — your annoying friend — urging you to schedule ten important health screenings we all need to undergo to remain strong and healthy. If your children needed these tests you would NEVER PUT THEM OFF. Well, your children need *you*.

Blood Pressure Test: Generally, when I first get my blood pressure taken at the beginning of a doctor's appointment, it tends to read high. I usually tell the nurse that I was probably just a little anxious and recommend that we try again at the end of the appointment. I've come to learn that there is something called *white coat syndrome,* where one exhibits a higher than normal blood pressure level, just by being in a medical setting.

This test is one of the most important because high blood pressure, also known as hypertension, usually has no symptoms. It can't be detected without being measured, and high blood pressure can greatly increase our risk of heart disease and stroke. The doctor or nurse will usually tell you what your blood pressure reading is on that day, but it's important that you ask what those numbers mean, and if they are not normal, what actions you should take to improve them.

Cholesterol Screening: This test, which involves a blood draw, measures two different types of cholesterol often referred to as our "good" and "bad" cholesterol. Our HDL (good) cholesterol helps prevent LDL (bad) cholesterol from clogging our arteries.

A typical cholesterol screening also measures our triglycerides, a type of fat found in our blood. A normal triglyceride level is

160

less than 150. Nearly 1 in every 2 American women has high or borderline high cholesterol. High cholesterol can lead to fat deposits in our arteries, which, in turn, can increase our risk for heart attack and stroke. So these are important numbers to watch, especially since we can take action to bring elevated cholesterol under control once we discover it. Your doctor can advise you on what to do so be sure to ask. Also, if you have high blood pressure or high cholesterol, talk to your doctor about whether you need a test for diabetes as well.

Gynecological Exam and Pap Smear: I don't know about you, but I love these — just kidding. I don't think any of us love having this test, but it's critical for our health. A gynecological exam can detect any abnormalities in the reproductive organs. A Pap smear is used to find either cell changes or abnormal cells in the cervix. Cells are lightly scraped or brushed off the cervix and sent to a lab. If detected early, cervical cancer can be cured. A woman's risk of cancer increases with age, so it is especially important for menopausal and postmenopausal women to continue their gynecological care to aid in early detection.

161

Mammogram: While this boob-squishing experience is often uncomfortable, it is the best way to detect breast cancer while it is most treatable. There has been a lot of debate over *when* we should begin our mammogram screenings and *how often* we should get them, but physicians I know feel there should be *no debate*. They recommend we begin our screenings at age 40 and get mammograms every year thereafter. Note that the American College of Physicians (ACP) and the U.S. Preventative Task Force tell us to wait until we're 50 and to only be screened every 2 to 3 years if we are at normal risk and have no symptoms. *I feel compelled to tell you about this only because I am so troubled by it.* If I had followed those recommendations, I would likely not be alive today to write this book. If there is a history of breast cancer in your family, you should get your first mammogram 10 years before the age your relative was diagnosed. If you have very dense breast tissue or a family history, you must be sure to talk with your physician about when you should begin screening and if you should also have an ancillary test such as an ultrasound or MRI.

Head-To-Toe Melanoma Skin Exam:

This is another one of those important screenings that women tend to put off because it requires getting naked and letting a doctor look incredibly close-up at every inch of our body. Okay, I agree, it's not my favorite exam either, but this important annual screening detects skin cancer, which is the most common cancer in America. The good news is that is a *preventable disease*. While more than 3 million cases are diagnosed each year, early detection often means it can be treated on an outpatient basis. Still, 9,000 people in the U.S. die from it. The deadliest form is melanoma. Although this kind is found in only 1 percent of all skin cancer patients, it accounts for 90 percent of all skin cancer deaths. Being vigilant about screening for skin cancer in general, and melanoma specifically, can save lives.

Some women find that they are more comfortable with a female doctor for this exam. But just remember, doctors do this all day. They are *not* judging our cellulite or unshaven legs. They are looking at our skin with the intent of keeping us alive longer.

Blood Sugar Test: This test checks for our risk of diabetes. Eighty-six million American adults in the U.S. are prediabetic — and 90 percent of them don't know it. That's just plain scary. Prediabetes means that our blood sugar levels are elevated, putting us at risk for diabetes, which can lead to heart disease, chronic kidney disease, stroke, vision loss, amputations, and even death. If the test shows we are prediabetic we can make simple changes in diet and exercise to delay or prevent the disease.

Colonoscopy: This test detects colon cancer, which is the third most common cancer in women. With a colonoscopy, colon cancer can almost always be caught when it is most curable — before symptoms even develop. For years doctors recommended that screenings begin at age 50 unless there is a family history of colon cancer, in which case screenings should begin ten years earlier than the age at which the relative was first diagnosed.

In response to a rise in colorectal cancer among younger people, the American Cancer Society recently began recommending that adults at average risk begin screening at age 45. In looking for factors that contributed to the alarming increase in this type of cancer among young Americans, researchers at the MD Anderson Cancer Center point to such factors as the rising rates of obesity, a lack of exercise, and the consumption of processed foods. It's long been known that diet plays a role in one's risk for colon cancer. In fact, the American Institute for Cancer Research says that good nutrition can reduce the incidence of many types of cancer by up to 40 percent.

> "Having a colonoscopy is the only time when 'What an asshole' would be considered a compliment."
> — UNKNOWN

Bone Density Test: This test is the only test that can detect the thinning of our bones, a condition known as osteoporosis. Since women are at greater risk of having this condition, which makes our bones fragile and more likely to break, all women age 65 and older should be checked for it. If your mother had it before you, or if you are light-boned and very fair skinned, or you've had a prior fracture, you should have this test to determine your bone density and to track how it changes over time.

Eye Exam: The reason an eye exam is so vital is that it can detect age-related changes such as macular degeneration, cataracts, or glaucoma. Doctors advise that between the ages of 40 to 65 we get tested every 2 to 4 years, and after age 65, every 1 to 2 years. If we wear glasses or contacts, we should have our eyes examined every year no matter how old we are.

Hearing Exam: untreated hearing loss has been linked to decreases in cognitive function, and increases in the likelihood of dementia, isolation, and depression. Discovering and treating hearing loss sooner rather than later can not only improve our overall health, it can enhance our overall enjoyment of life. A lot of people wait until they are having difficulty hearing before getting tested, which means they may have been living with hearing loss and its effects for years or even decades

So here's the *bottom line:* It's up to us to get our *tushies* to every appointment so we can be sure to have these life-saving tests. Although that pun was intended, this is serious business. The kind of vigilant self-care I've just outlined is what gives us the potential to stave off illness and live longer, healthier lives.

It's never too late to take control of your health!

For decades, we've been taught to be obedient, compliant patients, always deferring to doctors and never questioning their findings or recommendations. But in today's environment, we need to become full-fledged partners in our health management. We must speak up and ask questions. There are so many new treatments for diseases and chronic conditions coming to the market at record speed that second, and even third, opinions are often warranted. And at a time when people are worried about financing health care treatment, shouldn't we put an emphasis on preventative care — which could actually help lower health care costs?

Certainly, the time has come to change the way we view our role in our own health care. I believe that if every one of us took this more empowered approach, we could improve health care and lower death rates considerably.

CHAPTER 10
THINK LIKE A DOCTOR

"The greatest wealth is health."
— VIRGIL, ROMAN POET

Soon after I heard the dreaded words, "You have cancer," I found myself fielding a battery of questions about my family's medical history. I wasn't even sure how to answer ones about my grandparents, aunts, or uncles. I was stunned that I knew so little. I realized in that moment that I never sought out the information necessary to build a useful personal health history. It was particularly challenging as my family never lived near any of our relatives. This geographical divide prevented me from being part of family conversations about my relatives' health.

My grandparents on both sides lived well into their 80s and 90s, and while my mom suffered a minor heart attack in her late 50s, she too was almost 95 when she passed. I translated all of this to mean; *Hey, I've got great genes. I'm in the clear.*

Truth be told, I did hear that each of my parents had a sibling with Type 1 diabetes. That, along with my mom's heart attack, meant that I had a family risk factor both for diabetes and heart disease. For years, I simply chose to ignore those details. But having been diagnosed with a life-threatening disease, one which required me to work with a number of doctors in order to receive effective chemotherapy and radiation, I realized that I had better start thinking more like a doctor. I needed to start taking notes on my family's medical history, especially as it related to breast cancer, and I had better do it fast.

In today's world of specialists, it is up to us to become the glue that holds all the puzzle pieces together. We must make sure that our doctors know our full family health history so they can see the complete picture. In addition, we need to let them know what medications we take, when and why we've been hospitalized, what other medical conditions we may have, what tests have been run already, and what, if any, diagnoses have been made by other physicians.

I am old enough to remember a very different time in medicine when the family doctor knew all of this information because he or she was probably treating all our relatives. My dad was one of those family doctors — he treated entire families.

I was only 13 years old when I unexpectedly lost my father in a plane crash, so I never had the opportunity to get to know him as an adult. A few years ago, however, I decided to learn more about him and what it was like to practice medicine back in the 1930s, '40s, and '50s. I reached out to several doctors and nurses who were his peers for their reflections on his life and legacy.

I began my inquiry by returning to my hometown of Sacramento, California, where my dad had started his career as a small-town physician and where he later spearheaded the building of a much-needed community hospital. Several of his colleagues described him as more than a doctor. They said he was a missionary of sorts, that it never mattered to him if a patient didn't have the means to pay. "It was all about making the person whole."

One doctor, Dr. James Reece, who had shared an office with my dad for years, told me that my father regularly made house calls, which in those days cost $5. He said that when it came time to leave the patient's home, my dad would not only write the needed prescription and leave it on the bed stand, he'd also leave money to cover the cost of the medication if he knew the patient couldn't afford it.

Another doctor told me that office visits were $2 in those days, but if a patient couldn't pay and refused to accept free care because of pride, my dad would find a project that needed to be done around our home so they could come on a weekend and work side-by-side with him once they were well.

Dr. Marvin Klein, a Sacramento gynecologist who often referred patients to my dad for surgery, told me a story about a patient of his who had developed a vascular condition that surely meant she would lose a leg — or worse, that she would die. There were no vascular surgeons in Sacramento who were able to perform the needed surgery at that time, so Dr. Klein turned to my father for help.

Dr. Klein said that my dad had been following the career of Dr. Michael DeBakey, the renowned cardiovascular surgeon who, while still in medical school, invented the modified roller pump, a critical component of the heart-lung machine. My father placed a call to Dr. DeBakey at Baylor University in Houston, Texas, where he practiced and asked if Dr. DeBakey would allow my dad to follow him around for a week to learn more about vascular surgery and, in particular, about the surgical technique required to operate on Dr. Klein's patient.

DeBakey agreed. My dad flew there and learned the technique. He returned to Sacramento and performed the intricate vascular surgery that thankfully allowed the patient to live a full life.

Another physician told me a story about a patient of his who had troublesome varicose veins. He said my dad not only agreed to do the difficult surgery, but he went into his home workshop and made his own vein stripping instruments, which shortened the 8-hour surgery into a mere 2 hours. I didn't know that story, but I remembered that workshop.

In fact, I have my own story about that workshop. I used to sneak in to see all the tools and equipment. One day I found a kit for making casts, and I just couldn't resist trying it out. I made a cast on my arm from my hand up to my elbow. I soaked it in water and let it dry and harden. Uh oh. It was on my arm to stay. There was no getting it off! The weather was chilly, so I hid the cast from my parents under bulky sweaters for a few days. But my mom finally saw it. (It's hard to keep anything from moms.) My dad had to cut it off with a power cast cutter. Whoops. Sorry, Mom and Dad.

My father ultimately specialized in cancer surgery and worked closely with the American Cancer Society, speaking at medical conferences, and representing the U.S. at the 9th International Cancer Congress in Moscow, Russia, in 1961. I was always in awe of my dad's life and had hoped to follow in his footsteps. But that plan derailed the summer before I went away to college. I went to work in the hospital my dad had founded and discovered very quickly that my career could never involve needles and scalpels.

What I gained from this trip down memory lane with my father's former colleagues were not only priceless stories about my dad and who he was as a man, I also gained a better understanding of how the practice of medicine has changed over the years. It was a very different time; doctors knew their patients' personal stories and would consult with one another to give their patients the care that they needed. We live in a very different world today.

It has become a passion of mine to help lead conversations about how we can best

173

manage our health so that we can enjoy longevity and all the promise that our later years hold for us.

I think a lot of people leave their health and wellness in the hands of their doctors and never contemplate *their* role in staying healthy. When they visit their doctors, they likely spend an abbreviated amount of time with them. They watch their physician write a few notes about their health into *their* medical files before being told the doctor will see them again in a year.

We leave with a tiny appointment card in our hand while all that information about our visit remains in a digital file. Sure, we can access that data if we want to, as long as we set up our password-protected patient portal. But so few of us ever do. Unlike prior generations, we have all of these important details at our fingertips, but how many of us actually use them? How many of us are good keepers of our own medical history?

A month or two later, when we visit another doctor, we're asked to fill out a health questionnaire. Uh oh. We can't remember everything that was said in our last appointment and we find ourselves hard pressed to answer vital questions. Where's the password for that medical file when you need it?

Interestingly, in most homes you will find some sort of system for keeping necessary files. Whether it's in folders or a pile in the kitchen drawer, we probably have a place where we stash such important life documents. I know in our house we have a catchall file cabinet for everything from school calendars to instruction manuals on the care and maintenance of household appliances, local take-out menus, and of course, information on Bentley, our precious Goldendoodle, including his grooming and vet visits.

But here's my question for you — where is that file on *you*? That indispensable file for the care and maintenance of your body? If it doesn't exist, or it's somewhere in the cloud but you can't recall how to get to it, you are having a major life-threatening disconnect with your health and your longevity.

We need to think more like doctors. We need to track the medical information our various specialists are now helping us to maintain. We need to be the conduit between our different doctors, sharing that information with them all. We need to be able to readily access our personal health records (PHRs) on our computers and our phones. We need to connect all of our doctors' offices to it, and our local hospital system too.

By being an active participant managing our health information we will ultimately be able to reduce duplicate testing, avoid contradictory medications, and help our doctors better strategize our care and avoid medical errors. The trend toward specialization in health care that has been occurring for decades makes it imperative that we be the stewards of our own health management.

Each of us is like a cake baked from an old family recipe. The recipe includes a little of this and a little of that. Over time, some family members may have improvised and added new ingredients. Similarly, we may know we got our curly red hair from grandma and our prominent nose from our dad, but those aren't the only ingredients passed down over time. There are medical conditions, such as heart disease, cancer, and Alzheimer's, that may have been thrown into the mix.

Of course, not all diseases are *passed down.* In fact, 70 to 90 percent of disease risk is thought to be due to environmental exposure. But to fully understand our health risks, we should, at the very least, be aware of our family health history. It can be an important tool in defending ourselves against chronic illness and aging. By talking with our immediate family members, we can gather clues about our risk for specific diseases. By understanding these risks better, we are able to make better and more informed decisions regarding screening, prevention, and care.

Since my own diagnosis, I have heard from many women with breast cancer who only learned after their diagnosis that their mother, grandmother, or aunt had breast cancer because it was never discussed within the family. This was not uncommon in past generations. It wasn't that long ago that a woman who received such a diagnosis would decide to receive treatment in total secrecy, without even family members or close friends being told. However, we now know that keeping such a major medical secret from family members could prove deadly to future generations.

In my own case, while there was no history of the disease in my family, I wrongly assumed that made me immune when, in fact, less than 15 percent of women diagnosed with breast cancer have a family history of it.

As we get older and our health concerns naturally increase, the need to take ownership of our personal health information increases too. I've wised up and have been reconstructing my health history so it can guide me, my family, and my doctors going forward. Hey, better late than never.

To create your complete family health history, you should gather information as far back as three generations. This means you will need to talk with relatives including grandparents, parents, uncles, aunts, siblings, cousins, nieces, nephews, and so on. Ask about chronic conditions, past illnesses, cancer, heart disease, hypertension, diabetes, and any other medical crises. Ask for specifics including the age of the relative at the onset of the illness, and details regarding surgery or treatment.

To create your own personal health record (PHR), compile a complete account of your medical history including everything from the most basic childhood illnesses, allergies, immunization dates, medications you have or are presently taking, doctors you are seeing and any surgeries you've undergone.

It takes quite a lot of work and time to amass all of this information, including calls to prior doctors. Some will provide the information for free; others will charge a processing fee. Admittedly, as I've gathered information, I've sometimes needed further guidance from my doctors to help me understand it. I'm not going to sugarcoat it; this is a big undertaking. I'm still working on my PHR so that if I need medical attention, anyone overseeing my health will now know which doctor to call.

If you look online, you will find many downloadable forms to create a Family Medical History and a Personal Health Record. When you complete your personal health history it's a good idea to keep it on your computer and on your phone. It's also recommended that you print it and give a copy to a family member.

Having this on-hand can be very helpful when filling out medical forms or speaking with your doctor, but more importantly, it allows you to feel *in charge* of your health management.

Here's another helpful tip: Anytime you go to the doctor and they ask who you want your information sent to, include yourself on that list. Ask right then and there for a copy of your records. They are obligated to give it to you and in doing this, you will have your most current information handy.

CHAPTER 11
A HEART-TO-HEART
ABOUT YOUR HEART

"Dear Heart, Please stop getting involved
in everything. Your job is to pump blood,
that's it."

— UNKNOWN

When I was in my 20s, while I was out one
day with my mom, she began experiencing
signs of a heart attack. She was in her 50s
at the time and seemingly in good health.
We were getting our hair done when the
salon owner came to me saying my mom
was lying down in her office. She thought
my mom might be having a heart attack.
My mom was trying to make light of the
situation, saying we had errands to run and
she didn't want to spoil our afternoon. I'm
not sure if I was bold enough at that age to
challenge her, but fortunately other women
in the salon insisted she go right to the
hospital. It was a good thing they did,
because she *was* having a heart attack.

Thanks to those other women, my mom got the help she needed. As I've mentioned, mom lived to be 94 years old, so a heart attack does not have to mean a death sentence, however, *not* getting medical attention can.

My mom's reluctance to get help is not uncommon. The American Heart Association conducted a survey that asked women what they would do if they saw someone showing the signs of a heart attack. Over 90 percent said they would stop and help get that person the medical attention they needed. However, when asked what they would do if they were experiencing those same symptoms *themselves,* fewer than half said they would go to the hospital.

How could that be?

Well, they had to care for a child, pick their kids up from school, or get to the store so they could cook dinner. Women typically put the needs of others before their own, even when they are having chest pain! Unfortunately, more women die from heart attacks than men for one simple reason — we ignore the signs, so we don't get help.

One reason this happens is because the symptoms of a heart attack for a woman aren't as well defined as they are for men. Men typically experience the "Hollywood" heart attack — a stabbing pressure in the chest and pain in the arm. Women are more likely to experience less-defined symptoms that can seem almost flu-like, including nausea, vomiting, shortness of breath, and back or jaw pain. Unfortunately, these confusing symptoms lull women into thinking their discomfort is something else and will likely subside.

When talk show host Rosie O'Donnell found herself experiencing these symptoms, she said that she googled "women's heart attack symptoms" and even though the list she found matched her symptoms, she simply took an aspirin.

It wasn't until the next day that she went to the hospital because her symptoms hadn't stopped. Doctors removed a large blockage from her coronary artery before inserting a stent to keep the artery open. Thankfully, Rosie's story had a happy ending, but it was close, and she warns other women to know the symptoms that women experience and to get help quickly.

Actress Susan Lucci was in a boutique waiting for purchases to be wrapped when she experienced a tightening in her chest that radiated around her ribcage. She'd felt it several times during the preceding weeks, but she felt she was in phenomenal shape and had no family history of heart disease, so she, too, dismissed the signs. However, this time the pain became much worse. She described it as "an elephant pressing on my chest."

As it happened, she waited several weeks before checking things out. When she finally went to the hospital, doctors found blockages clogging nearly 90 percent of the artery that supplies most of the blood to her heart and 75 percent of another artery. A heart attack is a full blockage. She was lucky to have avoided that, but she still needed emergency surgery to insert a stent into each damaged artery. I know that, like me, she would encourage you under similar circumstances to seek immediate care to prevent a potentially fatal heart attack.

Although we women tend to put off getting care for ourselves, we should consider the fact that we'd never consider putting off proper medical treatment for our children. The first sign of a sniffle or cough, and off to the doctor we go. And don't we all nag our mates to get regular checkups? Yet we are notorious for not putting ourselves on our own to-do list.

I know this from personal experience. Two years ago, I found myself having some of these symptoms. I was actually sitting in a doctor's office waiting for my husband, who was having a colonoscopy. I'd been feeling fluish for several days, but I kept going. I even continued to work out because, you know, it was probably nothing. Right?

On that day, I was present as a wife, not a patient. Isn't there some kind of unwritten rule that only one spouse can be sick at any given time? I was supposed to be the caregiver that day, but I awoke feeling worse than the day before and was also experiencing pain up and down my left arm. I'll admit, I really started worrying. More than once I almost asked the nurse to take me into an exam room and do an EKG. But I didn't. Why? It was almost as though I was frozen with fear that something might really be wrong. The longer I sat there, the more I argued with myself. *Come on, don't be a baby. I probably just have the flu, right? But what if it was really a heart attack? How could I just assume it was not? It happened to my mom, so it seemed feasible it could be happening to me. Was I being irresponsible? I was there to take care of Jeff. Being there for him was my role that day. Who would drive him home after his procedure if I was having a heart attack?* These were the thoughts running nonstop through my head.

When my husband's procedure was finished, we drove home and I had him lay down so the anesthesia could wear off. I joined him on the bed, closed my eyes, and tried my best to ignore how I was feeling. However, an hour later when Jeff started feeling better, I was still feeling the same symptoms. I knew I had to say something. I began by telling him that I probably just had the flu, but that I had been experiencing symptoms all day that could also be a heart attack. "Jeff, you know I stand before audiences all the time telling them more women die of heart attacks than men because we don't go for help. I can't make that mistake myself! If I don't go to the hospital and get checked out, I'll be the biggest hypocrite."

We immediately went to the emergency room at our local hospital. Again, I prefaced my description of my symptoms to the ER staff by saying, "It's probably nothing — likely just the flu." But when I told them what I had been feeling they immediately treated it as a cardiac event, giving me an EKG, taking my blood pressure, a chest X-ray, and a battery of blood tests. Eventually they did a flu swab and determined it was not a heart attack, but rather the flu, even though I had a flu shot months earlier. As for the arm pain, they said I likely strained my muscles because I kept working out when I was so fatigued. (Oops. My bad.)

As soon as I heard that it was only the flu, my immediate reaction was to apologize profusely to the ER personnel for needlessly taking up their time. The ER doctor and the cardiologist were quick to assure me that considering my symptoms, I had made the right decision to get checked out. They said if more of us acted on our symptoms, there wouldn't be as many women dying from heart attacks.

We, as women, are very instinctual. We know when something is wrong. We must listen to and honor our intuition and our bodies, and never assume that worrisome symptoms will just pass. That is what ends up killing too many women.

We Need to Be Heart Smart

Now is as good a time as any to have a real heart-to-heart conversation with you about why and how you must protect your heart. Are you ready for a statistic that will blow your mind? An estimated *42 million American women* are living with cardiovascular disease, and many are completely unaware of the threat they face.

Heart disease is the leading cause of death for women in this country, with more than

200,000 women dying each year from heart attacks. That's five times the number of women who die from breast cancer!

The best way we can protect ourselves from heart disease is not only to know our family history but to know how it affects our individual risk. That means discussing it with our doctors. We also need to *know our numbers.* That means our blood pressure, cholesterol, resting heart rate, blood sugar levels, and our BMI (that stands for body mass index and is a measurement of our body fat based on our height and weight). I checked a BMI chart recently and decided that I'm just too short for my weight!

There's one more number that can reveal a great deal about our risk of heart disease . . . *our waist size.*

I don't know about you, but the only person who has ever measured my waist is a seamstress. I'm really good about going to my annual exams, yet no doctor or nurse has ever mentioned it. They've put me on the scale — but my waist? Nope. That has never happened. I asked a group of women ranging in age from their 50s to their 80s whether they had ever had a doctor measure their waist size during an exam. All of them said no. If this is a key indicator of our health, how is it possible that none of the doctors with whom I've come into contact in my entire life have ever measured it? It seems to be a critical piece of information, and one that is so easy to come by. Some health experts say if we can only remember one number, believe it or not, our waist size would actually be the biggest indicator of heart disease.

The reason waist size is so important is because when excess fat is carried around the middle (as opposed to around the hips or elsewhere) it can be an indicator of internal fat deposits coating the heart, kidneys, liver, digestive organs, and pancreas, which can increase our risk of high blood pressure, high cholesterol, heart disease, and Type 2 diabetes. This risk goes up with a waist size that is greater than 35 inches for women, and greater than 40 inches for men.

In other words, when it comes to our health risks, *where* our fat is stored on our body is actually just as important as *how much* fat is stored on our body. So take a look. Do you think your body type is more like an apple or a pear?

Don't waste another minute without this pertinent information. It's not necessary to wait around for your doctor. You can measure your own waist; all you need is a tape measure. Start at the top of your hip bone and then bring the tape measure all the way around your body, level with your belly button. Make sure that it's straight and even in the back. Don't pull too tight and don't hold your breath while measuring. Check the number on the tape measure right after you exhale.

Some health professionals advise that we keep our waist measurement less than half that of our height. So if your height is 5' 4" (64 inches) we should keep our waist size under 32 inches. If our height is 5' 8" (68 inches) we should keep our waist size under 34 inches.

So what do you do if your waist size is larger than what is considered healthy? You can't spot-reduce your waist (or any other part of your body). Crunches will strengthen your abs, but to lose inches around your waist, it will mean eating fewer calories and burning calories with exercise.

For every 8.5 pounds you lose, you can reduce one inch off your waist. Losing even one inch can result in significant improvements in all the other heart health numbers.

A Risk Wrap-Up

As we end this little heart-to-heart, let's all ask ourselves the following questions. Be honest! Your life depends on it!

1. Am I overweight?
2. Have I measured my waistline?
3. Do I smoke cigarettes?
4. Do I have high cholesterol?
5. Do I live a sedentary lifestyle?
6. Am I positive I'm not diabetic or pre-diabetic?

If you don't know the answer to all of these questions, you need to see your doctor. Like, right now. Get this information and make some decisions based on what you find.

Many women can significantly reduce their risk of heart disease if they have the information they need, get regular check-ups and screenings, and know what questions to ask during their doctors' appointments.

Okay, gotta go. Have to measure my waist.

"Suck it up, and one day you won't have to suck it in."

— Unknown

Chapter 12
Keep Moving! It's Harder for the Undertaker to Catch Up With You

"If you think a minute goes by really fast, you've never been on a treadmill."

— Unknown

I don't know about you, but I'm finding it harder these days to get my energy up to work out. Even when I'm in the gym, I don't always have the oomph to do one more set. I'm often wondering whether I've just hit a plateau, if it's my mindset that day, *or* if it's simply a matter of aging. The truth is, I sometimes need new ways to motivate myself. I'm always looking for alternate workouts to take away the drudgery that sometimes comes with exercise. Boredom in the gym is the worst. When I find an activity that's fun, I look forward to doing it again. Keep changing up your exercise routine and you'll never tire of it.

If you've been slacking off, or if you don't even have an exercise routine, then pay attention. *There's no disputing the evidence — adding any type of exercise to our day is a necessity for women as we age.* Aerobic exercise is crucial for maintaining cardiovascular and brain health, while resistance training helps maintain our muscle mass and increases our bone density. What's more, Harvard researchers say regular exercise decreases our risk of death from *any* cause by nearly one-third.

Physical activity also helps relieve stress and beat depression by releasing happy chemicals known as endorphins. And did I forget to mention that it helps us fit into our clothes too? I don't know about you, but *that* gives me happy endorphins!

And hey, I'm not talking about running a marathon, although, if you are running marathons, or even 5Ks, kudos to you! I would never get up on a pulpit and tell you to do something that I wouldn't do. Or your doctor doesn't recommend for you. Candidly, I'm more of a Zumba/weight-training girl than a runner. In my dreams I'm a runner; you should see me . . . I'm fast.

> "I named my dog Five Miles so I can say
> I walk five miles every day."
> — UNKNOWN

Seriously, daily exercise may be the closest thing we have to a fountain of youth. Even moderate exercise — a brisk 30-minute walk each day — can lower our risk of heart problems. And it's believed that regular high-intensity exercise, such as running, can possibly add up to four years to our life.

According to the Mayo Clinic, during aerobic activity where we repeatedly move large muscles in our arms, legs, and hips, the following happens:

- We breathe faster and more deeply, which maximizes the amount of oxygen in our blood.
- Our heart beats faster, which increases blood flow to our muscles and back to our lungs.
- Our small blood vessels widen, also delivering more oxygen to our muscles and carrying away waste products such as lactic acid.
- Our body releases endorphins, natural painkillers that promote an increased sense of well-being.
- And finally, exercise also improves the blood flow to our brain, which has been associated with a significantly reduced risk of Alzheimer's disease.

Okay, now I really got your attention! And you're sitting up at least (rather than reclining). I mean, that's something; a *very* little something but, nevertheless, you are *alert* and that's great.

It's not that we don't know we need to exercise. *Of course* we do. It's just that most of us don't follow through. A study by the American Heart Association shows that 75 percent of American women say they embrace the concept, but less than 25 percent say they're actually engaging in enough physical activity to make a significant difference in their health. In this crazy, hectic world of ours, how is it possible that women can do just about anything, but we can't figure out how to schedule exercise into our lives?

I think this is a real sticking point for a lot of us. We want to nourish and care for our bodies, but it can sometimes be perplexing to find the time or the compelling enough activity to get us to the gym on a regular basis. If we don't find an activity we actually enjoy, we'll never keep it up.

As I mentioned, my husband owns and operates summer camps in Maine, where we spend three glorious months a year. During that time, I work out with a fitness trainer, Beth Bielat, who has become a good friend and who has had a profound impact on my life. She's tiny in form but huge in energy, both physical and spiritual. She kicks my butt with a big smile on her face, and she tells me what I need to hear, not what I want to hear. That makes her a good friend in my book.

Beth helped put together a group of women who work out with me during those summer months. We are all fortunate to have her as our trainer and personal wellness guru. Beth may not realize it, but she has gone way beyond making us more fit; she has challenged us to honor our bodies and our souls in a subtle yet fierce manner. She's helped us all approach working out as an incredible opportunity to take our fitness to a new level. She constantly changes up our workouts so that we remain committed. We work till we're sweaty and we laugh till we . . . well, more about that later.

A few summers ago, Beth introduced our group to HIIT training. At first when I heard about this, I thought it meant I could "hit" her whenever she pushed us and we were tired. Yeah, it turned out that's not what she meant. HIIT training has proven to be quite helpful in losing weight, since we continue burning fat long after we stop the workout. It can also be valuable in delaying aging. In fact, experts now say that it could actually reverse some of the cellular signs of aging. Clearly, you can see why we're so excited about it.

HIIT training calls for short, quick blasts of very intense movement followed by a brief period of rest. In my workout classes we do a form of it called Tabata. It has become a staple in my fitness regimen. If you google it, you'll find lots of workout variations set to different genres of music. I've downloaded several of them and love the easy call-outs: "Get ready, prepare . . . and work . . . 20 seconds later; three, two, one and . . . rest. Cycle one complete." You simply follow the recorded commands and do eight sets of eight different exercises. It's pretty much a no-brainer workout set to awesome music. Here is a rundown of a typical Tabata session:

- Work out vigorously for 20 seconds (using either a strength or cardio exercise)
- Rest for 10 seconds.
- Repeat that exercise eight times. Then, you will have completed Cycle One.
- Do this with eight different exercises to complete eight rounds.

You want to push yourself as hard as you can for that 20 seconds of squats, lunges, or jumping jacks, and then when it's time to rest, come to a full stop for 10 seconds. You just keep repeating that sequence until you've completed eight sets.

We also do other HIIT classes with Beth that incorporate one-minute intervals with 30 seconds of rest in between. There are myriad interval training variations so you can find one that you like. They're hard but I think they're fun and suspect you will think so too.

Bear in mind, fat burn is greater when exercise intensity is higher. For years there has been a strong focus on calories burned during exercise, but new research reveals that it is also important to focus on what happens after exercise is over.

By pumping such high quantities of oxygen into our system, HIIT workouts boost our metabolic rate for several hours, so we continue to burn calories long after the exercise is over. You gotta love that!

HISTORY OF TABATA TRAINING

Here's a little history of Tabata training. It was discovered by Japanese scientist Dr. Izumi Tabata and researchers from the National Institute of Fitness and Sports in

Tokyo. It was designed to help train top-performing speed skaters. Tabata and his team conducted research on two groups of athletes; one group trained at a moderate intensity level while the other trained at a high intensity level. The moderate intensity group worked out five days a week for a total of six weeks; each workout lasted one hour. The high intensity group, by contrast, worked out four days a week for six weeks; each workout lasted four minutes and 20 seconds, with 10 seconds of rest in between each set.

The results: Group 1 improved their *aerobic* capacity but showed little or no improvement in their *anaerobic* capacity. Group 2 showed increases in *both.* Their aerobic capacity topped Group 1's and their anaerobic capacity improved by 28 percent. (Aerobic exercise, as you may know, benefits the cardiovascular system, whereas anaerobic exercise builds muscle mass.) In conclusion, high intensity interval training has more impact on both the aerobic and anaerobic systems and helps you lose more body fat because it keeps burning calories long after the exercise session is over.

> "No matter how slow you go, you are still lapping everybody on the couch."
> — SUSIE MILLER

One of the secrets to making workouts more fun and engaging is finding workout buddies with the same desires and fitness goals. This has always been a great tactic for me, whether I am training for a mountain climb or just trying to keep in shape. These buddies are there to cheerlead me on and to guilt me when I try to slack off, and I do the same for them. Think about who in your circle of friends or workmates might want to take a boxing class, do yoga, meet up and take a power walk, or go on a hike. Who can you connect with to help you meet your goals? Not only is it a great way to see your friends, it makes exercise much more enjoyable.

My group of exercise buddies sings along to the music, tells stories, laughs — and yes, sometimes when one of us has a life crisis, we cry together. It's a communal experience that I wouldn't trade for the world. When we're not getting our butts kicked by Beth, we embark on hikes that we probably never would've taken on our own, but together we encourage one another to keep climbing, knowing that at the top of the mountain we will sit and look out at a beautiful Maine view and be so happy that we met the challenge — and one another. It's not only good for us physically, but I think connecting with nature is extremely important to us mentally and spiritually too.

Another tactic that got me moving again was recalling what activities I found fun when I was a child. I loved horseback riding as a kid, so when my eldest daughters took up equestrian sports, I decided to join in on the fun. I ended up competing in horse shows as an adult right along with my girls. I loved every minute of it; that is, until I fell off jumping a course and broke my shoulder. Have you noticed that the older we get, the harder the ground gets? Being in a sling for months, followed by several more months of physical therapy, tempered my future jumping dreams. That's when I decided to hang up my saddle for good. So I guess wild horses are the *only* thing that can drag me away from fitness.

Tennis was a sport I never played growing up, but one that I learned much later so I could join in on the fun with my husband and friends. The first time I picked up a racket, I was embarrassed that I needed beginner lessons. Most of the people I knew learned to play as kids and were very well practiced. I finally decided that if I wanted to be a worthy opponent for them, I'd have to get over my self-consciousness and work with an instructor.

I found one who specialized in teaching beginner adults. Whereas I might have been embarrassed if my husband had to teach me something as basic as lobbing the ball back over the net, I was able to freely learn with an instructor whose job was to be patient and non-judgmental. As it turned out, tennis is now one of my favorite activities. Having gotten over saying "Sorry" every time I catapult the ball over the net, my latest goal is to play well enough to hold my own in a league.

There was one other activity that had been on my wish list forever, but somehow eluded me, and that was hiking. It always seemed so adventurous, especially mountain climbing. My mom and dad weren't the camping and hiking type, so I was that adult who'd never pitched a tent or slept under the stars. Fortunately, when I was at *Good Morning America,* I worked out at a nearby gym where they were planning to take a group to Jackson Hole, Wyoming, to climb the Grand Tetons, so I signed up to go.

Yep, I really did it. I know. I surprised myself too. I think I registered while extremely sleep deprived and didn't fully understand what I was getting myself into!

I was 45 years old at the time and almost all the other climbers were in their 20s and 30s. Was I really going to do this? We trained for several months and then one evening our climbing group attended a mandatory meeting to hear about the terrain, the challenges, the possibility of altitude sickness, and the dangers of an avalanche. Whoa! Did they say avalanche? Seriously, as scary as that sounds, I bet right about now some of my menopausal friends reading this are dripping perspiration on the page and thinking being covered with snow sounds kind of nice right about now! LOL!

By the end of the meeting they handed out a list of the mountain gear that we would need, and after taking one look at it I began to think I was in over my head.

Items You Will Need for the Teton Climb
Waterproof/Insulated jacket, pants, and gloves *(Okay, they want us to stay warm and dry.)*
Waterproof hiking boots and hiking socks *(Sounded cozy enough to me.)*
Backpack *(What color should I choose?)*
Sleeping bag *(My daughters had some from sleepovers. Could I borrow one of those?)*

Headlamp *(Like, from my car??)*

Sun-shielding hat or cap, sunglasses, sunscreen, and lip balm *(Oooh, now these are some products I can get behind!)*

Water bottle and water treatment system with iodine tablets *(Excuse me?)*

Gaiters to be worn over your boot and lower pant leg to keep snow out *(Like, bell bottoms?)*

Carabiner *(Not to be confused with someone from the Caribbean. These are the small connectors for safety ropes so we don't fall to our death. Uh, did they say death?)*

Crampons *(No, it's not what you're thinking. Turns out, these are metal contraptions that look like bear traps. They attach to the bottoms of your hiking boots so you don't fall off the snowy mountainside. Once again, to your death?)*

Ice axe *(This is exactly what it sounds like. It's an axe. They asked me to bring an axe! Cue the banjos from* **Deliverance***! It was starting to feel a little "Lizzie Borden" to go axe shopping.)*

Toilet paper *(Uh oh, I'm starting to get the full picture here. How would I pack a supply of two-ply jumbo rolls? Would Amazon Prime deliver? They have everything; they* *must have Sherpas.)*

Our plan was to make it to the top of the middle Teton, which is an elevation of 12,805 feet. The climb to the summit is roughly two miles, but it ascends 2,700 feet and usually takes 6 to 8 hours to climb. Two dozen members of the gym were on the list for the mountaineering retreat. I had signed up for this journey with my good friend and colleague, Laura Morton, who had produced a workout video with me following my very public weight loss and has since co-authored three books about my journey to fitness and my breast cancer survival story. But on an extreme adventure like this one, we were about to find out how healthy and fit we really were.

In the weeks leading up to the big event, we prepared by power walking on gym treadmills with the backpacks we would be using on the climb. The treadmills were set to the highest incline and the gym's owner — our fearless leader — walked around adding more to our backpacks to make them increasingly heavy.

When the day finally arrived, I met my fellow climbers at LaGuardia Airport where we boarded a flight to Jackson Hole, Wyoming. It was June and a magnificent sunny morning when we started the trek up to our base camp. We were only going from 6,000 feet to 8,200 feet that first day, and it was estimated that it would take four hours. How hard could that be? Well, within the first hour we had to change into hard shell hiking boots and those gaiters that were on the packing list to deal with the snow.

As the day wore on, the temperature kept dropping while the grade kept rising, getting steeper and steeper. I wondered whether the younger climbers were worried about their endurance, their breathing, and their heart rate, because I sure was. The scenery was *breathtaking.* Yes, I used that word purposely.

When we finally arrived at our destination for the day, we found a small village of tents set up. I slipped into mine and found that when I laid on my sleeping bag, my head sloped more downhill than my feet. After 30 minutes in that position, I began to feel a little woozy.

At dinnertime, we all sat around on what looked like a topless igloo. Seriously, it was a big round seat of cold compacted snow. They handed me a bowl of soup, but the thought of eating made me nauseous. Altitude sickness was already setting in. Yuck. Fortunately, a GMA viewer had sent me climbing advice, which included a list of meds I should carry in my backpack just in case. Soon after dinner, we all returned to our tents so we could get a good night's rest for a full day of falling lessons the next day.

Yep.

Falling lessons.

Remember that ice axe I was told to purchase? Well, the next morning we put it to good use practicing every conceivable way we could fall down a 45-degree mountain and still catch ourselves. As grueling as this practice was, it sure beat falling to our death. They called this technique *self-arrest*.

I called it *scary*.

Did I really sign up for this?

Sleeping on the icy cold mountain presented another bewildering problem. We had been encouraged to stay hydrated at that elevation, but as we all know, what goes in must come out. The challenge was that our outhouse was nothing more than a bucket hidden behind a tree . . . oh great, that's a good visual. But it still didn't answer the question, "Are we really going to put on our boots and cold weather gear to go out in the dark cold night to pee?" No way. So I devised a plan that could only be hatched by a female brain. I took stock of the supplies in my backpack and found that I had put my toiletries in small ziplock bags. I decided that these bags could be repurposed — meaning, I could pee in them! But then what? It was too embarrassing to discard those little baggies in front of the tent entrance, so I emptied them into the snow just outside. I laughed so hard I almost had to pee again. I really thought I was being so clever and resourceful! The only problem with that is I had emptied the bags next to the very spot where the tent was pitched, and the warm pee quickly melted the snow. You know where this is going — yep, the tent started to droop. Do you think the others noticed?

After the second night of sleeping on that icy mountain, we were awakened at 1:30 a.m. to begin our ascent to the top in nothing more than the dim light of the moon. At one point the guides had us stop to rest and eat a small snack, but mainly it was to watch the sunrise and take pictures. As the horizon glowed before us, the wind picked up and then the rain came. Ugh! But we just kept climbing.

As soon as the downpour stopped, we encountered a field brimming with rocks and boulders that were incredibly hard to navigate. It intimidated us all.

When we finally reached the summit after climbing for almost ten hours, I was so exhausted and frozen that it was hard to get excited even though there in Wyoming I had a magical view of Idaho to my right and Montana to my left. The wind that high up almost blew me over. My tired body was already feeling like a bit of a rag doll.

I said, "Okay, it's amazing, now let's go." Standing there on top of the world, all I could think was, "How in heaven are we going to get back down this mountain?"

The answer: Not easily.

During our training we had been taught that people were more likely to get hurt on the way *down* the mountain than they were on the way *up.* Now I know why. When you're freezing and totally exhausted, the determination and drive you once had to reach the summit is nearly gone. You pretty much just want it to be over. As the afternoon temperatures plummeted, the snow began to harden so that each time we took a step, our boots aggressively crunched through the top layer of ice and then slid down into the soft snow beneath. A recipe for disaster.

The climb leaders soon realized that our small group had lagged and that we were behind schedule (aka, they realized that we might need some extra care on the way down so that we wouldn't kill ourselves!). As the first order of business, they linked us all together with ropes and those carabiners so that if any one of us began to fall uncontrollably on the steep mountain, the rest of the group would be able to secure themselves with their ice axe and catch the fall. By the way, that happened. My friend Laura lost her footing and fell. In an instant, she started slipping on the icy surface right off the edge of the mountain. Believe it or not, it was me who flew into action burying my axe deep into the ice so we could stop her from falling. Drinks were on her that night, but seriously, we've had each other's backs ever since.

Climbing the Tetons is good cocktail party talk these days, but candidly it turned out to be a whole lot harder than I ever expected. But I will say that it was much more meaningful than I had ever imagined too. It made me push myself so far beyond what I thought my limits were, and in the end the Teton adventure expanded my idea of how much I can expect of myself and of my life. It also taught me another valuable lesson. As we stood on the mountain that morning, it was clear that a few of us weren't going to make it to the tallest peak. Our guide simply told us to look around, because there were peaks *everywhere.* We didn't need to summit the *highest* peak to get to the top of one. He said, "Pick your peak." And that's exactly what we did. From that day forward, I took that lesson with me and have used it as a guiding light whenever I am making tough decisions.

That experience energized me and lent me the courage to try other adventures that involved snow, ice, and mountains. It had been years since I'd gone skiing, but after our twins were born, I was so much more confident taking them to the slopes to get them acclimated to the great outdoors. By the way, it took them about 30 minutes before they were ready to go to the top of the chair lift. No fear. They just followed the classic beginner's advice and made their skis form *pizza slices* and *French fries.* In no time they were zooming down the mountain like they'd skied their whole life.

Now listen, I'm not saying you have to climb a mountain. I'm just suggesting that you step outside of your comfort zone. You can choose and design your own adventure. The point is to find something that excites you.

If you can, get your whole family involved. Ski together, hike together, and play ball in the backyard. This infuses a sense of fun and play into family time and it also sets a good example for the kids. If children grow up expecting that sports and fitness are a natural part of life, they will be way ahead of the health game as adults.

"Don't expect to see a change . . . if you don't make one."

— UNKNOWN

CHAPTER 13
WE'RE BASICALLY A HOUSE PLANT WITH MORE COMPLICATED EMOTIONS: WHY WE NEED WATER

"You know you're getting old when you can't walk past a bathroom without thinking, 'I may as well pee while I'm here.' "

— UNKNOWN

Did you know that a human can go for more than three weeks without food but can only last a few days without water? That fun fact kind of floored me when I first heard it. Mostly because I can barely go a day without food. And I might as well confess right here at the beginning of this chapter that I've never been great at hydrating. So, there you have it. I'm just not a good water drinker. I find consuming the recommended 6 to 8 glasses of water a day torturous. And I don't think that I am alone. When I was diagnosed with breast cancer and started chemotherapy, I was told it was imperative that I drink 8 to 10 glasses of water daily as some of the side effects of chemo can cause dehydration. *Uh oh. Now what?*

I was lousy at getting in the daily allotment when I wasn't in the fight of my life, so how could I possibly do it to survive chemo? I was also aware that whenever someone asked me how many glasses I'd consumed on any given day, I'd grossly overexaggerate! Not just because I was trying to pull one over on whomever was asking, but because I really thought I'd been better at it. But now that there was so much at stake, I had to get serious. After all, the only person getting hurt by the lack of hydration was me!

I think many of us feel there's nothing more boring than a plain old glass of water, but of course I've learned that water serves a much bigger purpose than simply quenching our thirst. For years I had never thought of water as a nutrient, even though it is actually one of the most critical nutrients in our diet. Every system in the human body counts on water to function.

About two-thirds of the adult human body is made of water. It comprises 85 percent of our blood, 75 percent of our brain, 90 percent of our lungs, 70 percent of our muscles (including our heart), 30 percent of our bones, and 64 percent of our skin. If we were a state, we'd be Michigan, surrounded by the Great Lakes!

In reality, most of us drink less than *half* the amount of water we're supposed to on a daily basis. And depending on what we're doing and where we are, we may need even more than the daily recommendation. Even if we spend more time in the lounge chair than swimming laps or playing tennis, we're still losing enough water each day to fill eight or ten glasses.

All of us lose water through our breath, perspiration, urine, and bowel movements. For our body to function properly, we must replenish its water supply by consuming beverages and foods that contain water.

The National Academies of Sciences, Engineering, and Medicine determined that an adequate daily fluid intake is:

About 15.5 cups (3.7 liters) of fluids for men

About 11.5 cups (2.7 liters) of fluids a day for women

Whether we are aware of it or not, water continually sneaks out of our system without us noticing. It doesn't just escape through sweat or saliva; we even lose some water just by exhaling. Other factors that can impact our hydration include:

214

- **Altitudes & Climates:** If we live in or are visiting a hot, humid, or dry climate or a location at a high altitude, our water needs might increase.
- **Indoor Variables:** If we are breathing dry air from a heater, dehumidifier, or air conditioner, our fluid loss can dramatically increase.
- **Sunbathing:** Lying in the sun increases our water loss due to perspiration. On a hot day, sweat can evaporate quickly, so just because our skin is dry to the touch doesn't mean we're *not* sweating. And remember, if we get a sunburn, we've most likely had increased water loss.
- **Exercise:** When we exercise, we can lose an enormous amount of water through sweating, which then needs to be replaced. An hour of working out can cost us one to two quarts of water, which means we'll need to double our daily water intake. Yikes! Being well hydrated enables our muscles to work longer and harder before tiring and this can help us build even more muscle. Drinking water also lubricates our joints and prevents muscle cramping. My calf muscles often cramp at night, so this is important to me.

- **Plane Travel:** Flying on an airplane can also induce water loss: during a three-hour flight we can actually lose one-and-a-half pints! I fly a tremendous amount, so I've created a water challenge to help me meet my goal to stay hydrated, especially on longer flights. I buy one of those tall 32-ounce bottles of water before boarding the plane and attempt to drink it all before I land. Completing the challenge means I've consumed four of the eight glasses recommended daily. Voila! And then I sprint to a bathroom upon deboarding.
- **Sickness:** Our body loses fluids when we have a fever, diarrhea, or vomiting. Other conditions that can require us to increase our fluid intake include bladder infections and urinary tract stones. In fact, water can help us avert UTIs and kidney stones altogether. Good hydration helps prevent crystals from sticking together and forming pesky stones. Water also helps dissolve the antibiotics used to treat urinary tract infections, making them more effective. Drinking more water also produces more urine, which flushes out bacteria.

A lot of us walk around in a state of chronic dehydration and don't even know it. I am one of them. And if we wait until we're thirsty to drink, it is kind of like waiting to gas up our car until the needle is on empty. By the time we feel thirsty, we're already dehydrated and that can leave us feeling fatigued.

Dehydration can cause headaches and constipation. When we drink sufficient water, it keeps everything moving through our gastrointestinal tract and thus prevents constipation. This may be TMI, but water helps dissolve waste particles so they can pass smoothly through our digestive system. When we are dehydrated, our body will pull water from our stools in order to maintain some hydration, and that will leave our colon dry, making it more difficult to poop. As long as we're in the bathroom, drinking plenty of water also prevents fluid retention, since our body won't try to retain water if it's already getting enough.

According to the National Sleep Foundation, being well hydrated can also determine how well we sleep. Their researchers found that if we go to bed dehydrated, it can influence our sleep patterns. Our dried-out nasal passages and mouth can increase the likelihood of snoring. Being dehydrated can also reduce our levels of essential amino acids, which are needed to produce melatonin, the sleep hormone.

Our brains are also impacted by how much water we consume. Keeping it well hydrated helps with our concentration and our memory function. When we are dehydrated, it can leave us feeling like our thinking is foggy and our moods are craggy.

Got a slow metabolism? Drink up! Seriously. Some recent research caught my eye. It showed that drinking a large, cool glass of water will increase your metabolism by up to 30 percent over a 90-minute period. I'll toast to that!

And finally, beauty really does come from within. When we drink water, we are hydrating skin cells, which plumps them up, making our skin look younger. Water moisturizes, replenishes tissue, and increases the elasticity of our skin. It also flushes out any impurities and improves blood flow, which can leave our complexion glowing. And that's what we want — healthy glowing skin! Water is more important than any lotion we'll ever buy. I guess the fountain of youth really is a fountain!

Chemo clearly taught me some lifelong lessons that have stayed with me to this day.

Here are some of the hydrating tips that really helped me — and are still helping me.

1. Add flavor to a big pitcher of water with slices of oranges, lemons, watermelons, or cucumbers.
2. Keep water with you at all times — a fresh bottle travels with me everywhere!
3. Drink water before and after workouts, though not too much during them.
4. Whenever you feel hungry, drink a glass of water instead of noshing. Thirst is often confused with hunger. The water also leaves me feeling full.
5. Schedule water breaks. I always drink water upon waking in the morning, before each meal, and a few hours before bedtime. While it's not good to go to bed dehydrated, I found that if I drink too close to bedtime, I'm up all night to pee. Give it some thought and create a schedule that works for you.
6. I actually have a high-tech water bottle that reminds me to drink. They're not called *smart* water bottles for nothing!

7. Now there are apps to help track your fluid intake.

Around the time I was getting chemo infusions, Beth Bielat taught another way to track my fluid intake. She got me some inexpensive thin plastic wrist bracelets that she ordered from the Oriental Trading Company. She told me to put ten bracelets on my right wrist and to move one of the bracelets to my left wrist each time I consumed an 8-ounce glass of water. This way I would be assured that I'd gotten the job done. It may sound simple, but it worked! All my girlfriends in my workout class did it with me. They agreed that they too found it difficult to keep track of how much water they actually drank, and this simple method was an ingenious way to monitor it.

Oh, and one more thing to keep in mind: If you fall behind, don't try to make it up by guzzling a lot of water during the evening hours. Take it from me, I did this a few times and let's just say I made too many trips to the loo to count on those nights. Bad plan.

As of the writing of this book, I am six years out from my cancer diagnosis, and I still struggle to take in the recommended amount of water each day.

As we age, our cells are constantly losing water. According to Dr. Howard Murad, who wrote *The Science of Cellular Water,* while 75 percent of our body is comprised of water when we are born, by the time we reach middle age, our body's water content can be as low as 50 percent. Cellular water loss causes aging, and our wellness is determined by each cell's ability to hold water. Without an adequate supply, our skin cell structure deteriorates and leads to fine lines and wrinkles. Dr. Murad says the ability of cell membranes to hold water is the fundamental marker of youthful good health and dewy skin.

I worked with Dr. Murad for ten years on one of his skincare lines and he always told me that I should *eat my water.* He said that when most people think of hydration, they think it just means drinking eight glasses of water a day, but that water will go right through you along with any nutrients. Dr. Murad emphasizes that hydration is about the water you are able to keep in your body, and the water in fruits and vegetables don't pass right through you. The water in fruits and vegetables is surrounded by molecules that facilitate the entry of water into cells, which is why it's called cellular water. This cellular water is absorbed slowly, thus providing us with lasting hydration. Dr. Murad says that while most foods contain some water, plant foods have more than other foods. He also tells us that when we consume water through fruits and vegetables, we are also getting antioxidants, anti-inflammatory agents, and fiber. Cooking vegetables reduces their water content so it's best to eat our fruits and veggies raw, blended, or juiced. Dr. Murad recommends the following.

Cucumbers: They're packed with potassium, which may help prevent a stroke. They also contain an anti-inflammatory substance called *fisetin,* which promotes brain health. It's one of the most hydrating foods, with a water content of 97 percent.

Strawberries: These are a favorite for smoothies. They have the highest water content of all the berries, 92 percent. Raspberries come in second at 87 percent, and blueberries are a cool third at 85 percent.

Watermelon: I love this juicy treat because it is filled with vitamins A, B6, and C, as well as lycopene and antioxidants. Eat it fresh, flavor water with it, or blend it into juice. Its water content is 92 percent.

Cantaloupe: This melon is a marvelous source of beta-carotene and vitamin C and also has a water content of 90 percent.

Grapefruit: Another great source of vitamin C, grapefruit has a water content of 91 percent.

Kiwis: Don't be fooled by a kiwi's size. They are not only packed with lots of water, they contain as much potassium as a medium banana and more vitamin C than an orange.

Peaches: According to researchers at Texas A&M, peaches have the potential to prevent obesity-related diseases such as diabetes and cardiovascular disease. And they're 88 percent water.

Carrots: Good for your vision and high in fiber, baby carrots are my mainstay snack. I love them with hummus. They have a water content of 87 percent.

Celery: This is a cancer-fighting superstar. University of Illinois researchers found that luteolin, a flavonoid in celery, has the potential to inhibit cancer cell growth especially in the pancreas. University of Missouri researchers found that apigenin, a compound found in celery, can stop breast cancer cells from multiplying and spreading. Also brimming with Vitamin A, this veggie has a water content of 95 percent.

Spinach: I use spinach in my morning smoothie. Its water content is 92 percent.

Broccoli: A nutritional powerhouse, this vegetable is filled with phytonutrients, antioxidants, fiber, vitamins, and minerals and has a water content of 91 percent.

Eggplant: It's low in calories and high in dietary fiber. Eggplants are also a good source of B vitamins, manganese, vitamin K, and potassium, which support our immune system and our cardiovascular system. Its water content is 89 percent.

Apparently, it not only matters *how* we take in our water, but *when* we take in our water. There is research that shows that we can absorb more of water's healthy benefits if we drink it at certain times. Conversely, there are also certain times when we should pass on water because our body is busy doing other things and needs a clear path to do so.

Drink up when you wake up: It is recommended that we drink our first glass (or two) of water on an *empty* stomach as soon as we wake up to help jumpstart our brain and body after sleep. High performance coach Brad Davidson suggests warm water with fresh lemon first thing in the morning, and yes, if you drink coffee, you should have that glass of water before your first cup of Joe. Apparently drinking two semi-warm glasses of water in the morning is a daily Japanese ritual that dates back to ancient times. The health, beauty, and longevity of the Japanese people have for centuries been attributed to this practice. Adopting this early morning routine can also help wash away any toxins and free radicals that have been hanging out in your circulatory system overnight. It can also clean and purify your body's internal organs. One further tip to bear in mind: Don't eat anything for 30 to 40 minutes after drinking the water, as that is how long it takes our body to cleanse.

Drink up before you chow down: Before any meal, be sure to drink a glass of water 30 minutes in advance. Doing this can help digestion. The water prepares our intestines for the food coming its way and can also help prevent us from overeating, since the water lines our stomach and makes us feel full. It's not wise to consume a lot of water during a meal or even immediately after eating. We absorb water best on an empty stomach and drinking a lot of it during or just after a meal dilutes the body's natural juices, which aid in digestion. This is not to say that we can't take small sips throughout our meals, since that can slow down eating and reduce our overall consumption.

Drink up before and after you work out: It's recommended that we have one to two glasses of water before hitting a gym so that we don't get dehydrated during our workout. Then after the workout, it's important to replace all the fluids that we lost through sweat. While you want to remain hydrated during a workout, it's not a good idea to drink too much since it can deplete our natural electrolytes and make us fatigued.

Drink up before a bath: This one didn't surprise me because I always find that a hot bath dehydrates me. Drinking one glass of warm water before our bath can promote dilation of our blood vessels, which helps lower our blood pressure. Consuming water also dilutes sodium in our body, which can further lower our blood pressure.

Drink up when you're worn down: Fatigue is a sign of dehydration. When we feel tired or when we have a big presentation coming up and need to be focused, we can fire up our brain by drinking a glass of water. Water moves quickly through our body and goes directly to our brain. By replenishing our brain's fluid levels, we increase our cognitive thinking.

Drink up before bedtime: Your body is busy repairing itself during the hours that you sleep, and your organs need to be well hydrated to get the job done right. If you find yourself getting up too many times during the night to pee, like me, then be careful of drinking too close to bedtime. Perhaps you can drink water in the early evening, setting a cut-off at an hour or two before you go off to sleep.

Don't drink up while standing up: I had never heard of this one before. Apparently, drinking while standing can have an adverse effect on our kidneys. Sitting while drinking allows our body to more efficiently filter the nutrients and then direct the water to those areas of our body that need nourishing, instead of going directly to our stomach with a force, as it does when we are standing. We also typically drink water a lot faster when we're standing, which can cause our nerves to tense up.

Finally, there is an easy way to check to see if we're drinking enough fluids and it doesn't take more effort than a trip to the bathroom. If we're drinking enough water, our urine will be pale yellow, which means we're well hydrated. Darker colored urine (particularly brown urine) can mean our body is crying out for more water.

I hope that these tips encourage you to hydrate more and that you take to the daily practice the way a duck takes to water — easily and naturally!

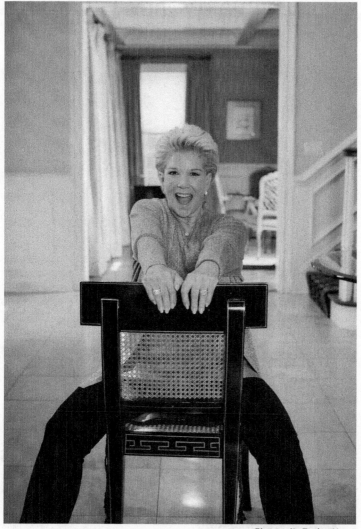

Aging can seem like a formidable opponent, especially for women.
But we can be prepared to tackle it head-on, and even enjoy it!

NOURISHING MY BODY AND BRAIN

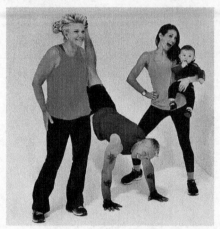

Photo credit: Daphne Youree

What's more fun than making exercise a family affair?! I am inspired daily by my daughter Jamie and her husband, George, who founded @NYCFitFam, here with one of their two children, Mason.

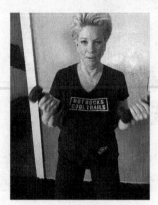

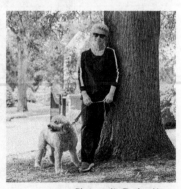

Photo credit: Daphne Youree

Always working on
maintaining t-shirt arms.

We can't forget to stop
and smell the roses…
or the pine trees.

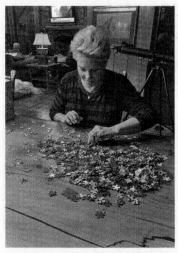

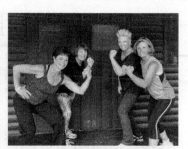

Friendship is one of the best Rx's for a happy life, especially as you age. Even better … working out with good friends!

My favorite brain challenge is a one thousand piece jigsaw puzzle. It's like playing a game of Concentration; I'm addicted to them.

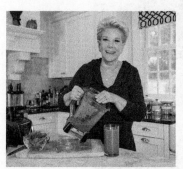

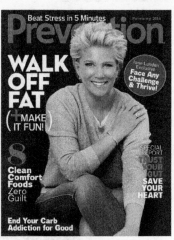

Photo credit: Daphne Youree

Photo credit: Courtesy of Prevention magazine, February 2016. Reprinted with permission of Hearst Magazines, Inc.

I'll admit, I prefer my avocado in guacamole, but it's also one of my favorite ingredients in my morning green smoothie!

Thank goodness I stepped up my powerwalk so I could fit into these jeans for the cover of *Prevention* magazine (one of my favorites).

BEHIND THE SCENES

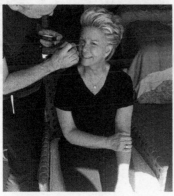

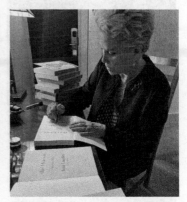

Hair and makeup stylist extraordinaire Emir Pehilj often accompanies me on the road for big events to work his magic before I step on stage.

I often check into a room filled with hundreds of books to sign before an event.

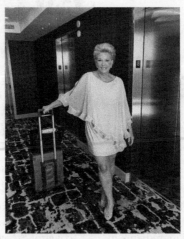

Hair and makeup ready and, as usual, with a suitcase in hand!

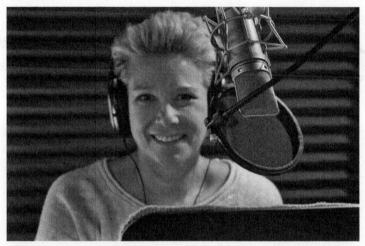

In the studio, recording the audio version of my book. (And if you're wondering… yes, headphones really ruin a good blow-out!)

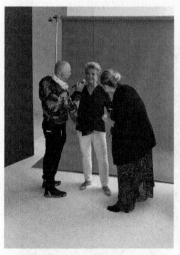

It takes a village to get the perfect picture.

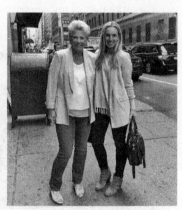

I'm lucky to have my daughter Lindsay work with me… whoever said "Don't mix family with business" didn't have as much fun as we have together!

MY LIFE ON THE ROAD

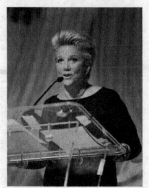

Photo credit: Sheri Whitko Photography

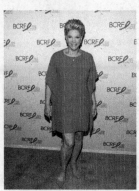

Photo credit: Rob Rich

There was a time when public speaking made me ridiculously nervous; now it's a favorite part of my career.

On the red carpet, or in this case, the pink carpet. I'm still trying to learn how to stand just right, so my legs look good! … a work in progress.

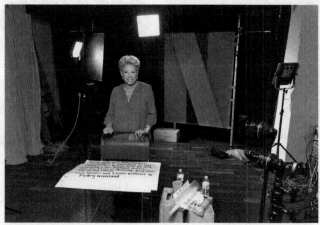

Getting ready for live interviews for a campaign I did with Netflix.

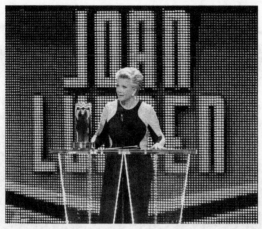

Photo credit: Courtesy of WWE

Big stage + clear podium = no short skirts!
(And by the way, that award was REALLY heavy!)

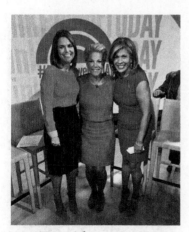

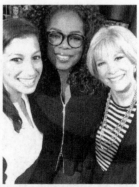

Two of the nicest and
brightest people on television,
Savannah Guthrie and Hoda
Kotb, on the set of *Today*.

When you're interviewed by
Oprah, you don't pass up the
opportunity to take a selfie with
her! Here, with my daughter
Sarah with whom I have also
gotten to work over the years.

THE LOVES OF MY LIFE

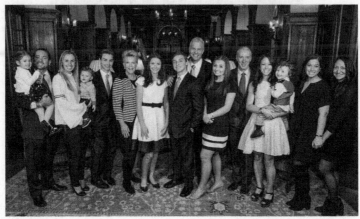

Photo credit: Frank Ammaccapane

With each big event, it seems our family grows!

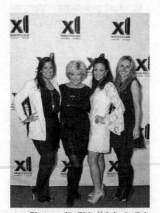

Photo credit: PMc // Sylvain Gaboury

I had my first three daughters, Sarah, Jamie, and Lindsay, while I hosted GMA; here they are all grown up on a NYC red carpet.

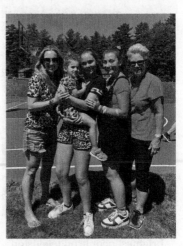

Showing our spirit on visiting day at one of my husband's summer camps, Tripp Lake.

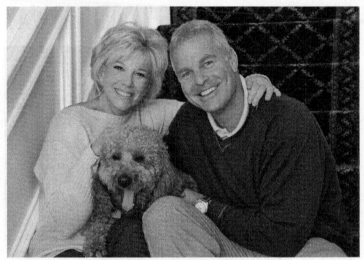

Snuggling with my favorite guy... and my
husband, Jeff (just kidding honey!).

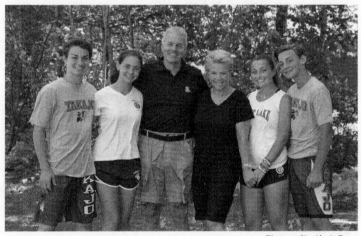

Photo credit: Alexia Berry

Surrounded by our twins Max, Kim, Kate, and Jack,
at Camp Takajo, Jeff's boys camp in Maine.

STRONG WOMEN WHO PAVED THE WAY

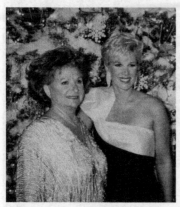

Celebrating Christmas at the White House, you can see why we always called my mom Glitzy Glady. (She loved this part of my job!)

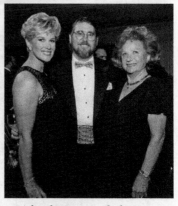

After losing my dad at age 13, my mom became our fearless leader, here with me and my brother, Jeff.

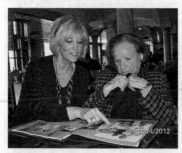

My mom loved looking at the the photo books I made about our life and her earlier years. She could talk about those early memories for hours. What she had for lunch 30 minutes ago? Not so much!

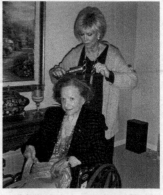

Old? Maybe… Well-coiffed? Absolutely! Keeping my mom "feeling like herself," even at 94 years old.

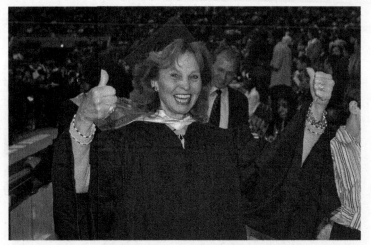

My mother-in-law, Janey, finally getting
her college diploma on her 70th birthday.

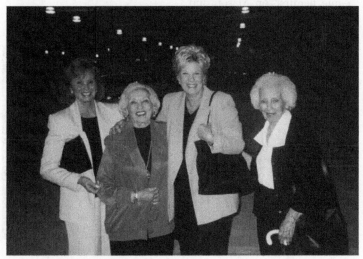

Family Matriarchs. Me with (from left) my mother-in-law,
Janey; her mother, Rosie; and Rosie's sister Millie. These
women have served as strong role models for our family.

MY LIFE AS JOJO

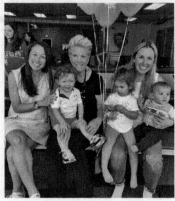

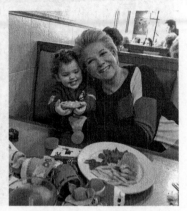

Life is always a party when you have grandchildren! (With Jamie, her first son, Mason, and Lindsay with Parker and Leo.)

The best lunch date ever! (Lindsay's son Leo)

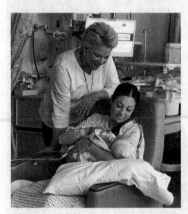

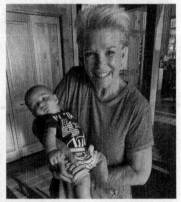

There is nothing more incredible than the birth of a new baby. (Jamie's second son, Asher)

Do I ever have to put him down? (Jamie's son Asher)

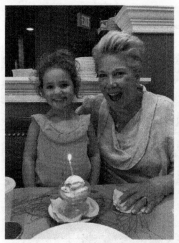

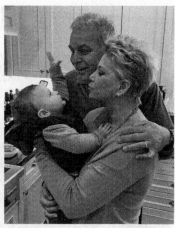

A party fit for a princess! Celebrating a birthday with our little Parker!

The best part about having grandchildren is that you can be as silly as you want! (Lindsay's son Leo)

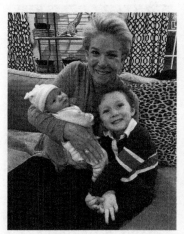

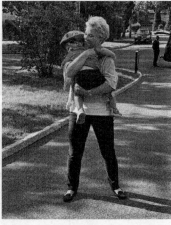

Mason is the best big brother to baby Asher.

Is there anything more delicious than a wraparound hug?! I don't think so! (Lindsay's son Leo)

AT HOME...

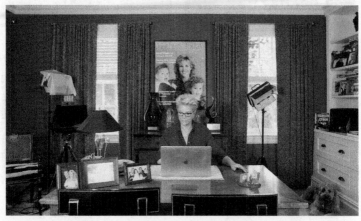

My home office also serves as a mini studio.

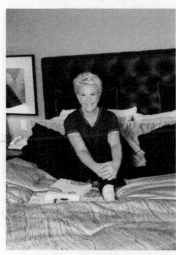

My bedroom is one of my favorite spots in my house.

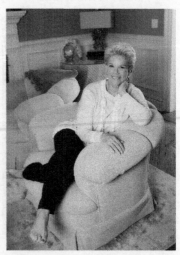

A silver lining of aging is finding contentment in relaxing at home.

ALL: Photo credit: Daphne Youree

AND EXPLORING THE WORLD
2001   2019

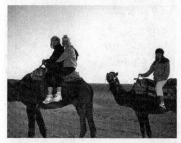

Sunrise over the Sahara

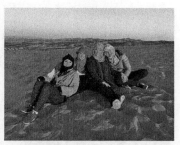

Same sand & sun, 18 years later

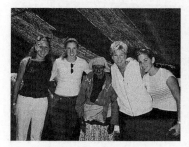

One way to get over the dunes…

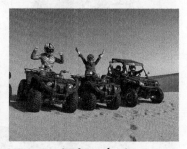

And another!

A woman who didn't
acknowledge her age…

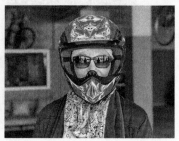

And another.

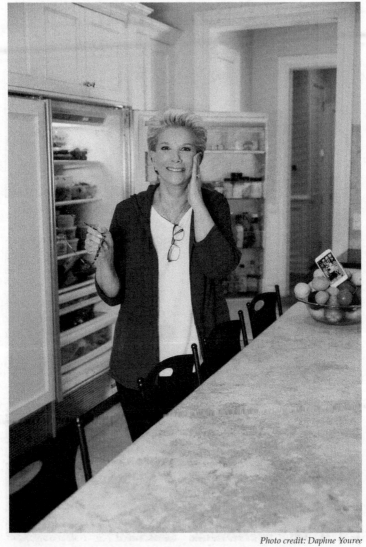

Why did I come into this room?!

Chapter 14
Sometimes I Laugh So Hard, Tears Run Down My Leg

"With age comes new skills . . . you can laugh, cough, sneeze, and pee all at the same time!"

— Unknown

Have you ever laughed or sneezed so hard that you . . . *leaked*? Don't worry, you don't have to answer that question aloud. But just know that you're certainly not alone. Leakage, or as your physician would call it, *urinary incontinence,* affects half of all women at some point in their lives.

Here's a new word of the day for you: *peezing.* It's a verb and it means sneezing and peeing at the same time. Try casually slipping this word into your conversation sometime and see the response. As I've grown older and my pelvic floor has become weaker, I've noticed that my aging bladder means business when it says, "I gotta go!" Seriously, it's almost as though our bladder is conditioned at a certain age to respond like a Pavlovian dog. If you ever took a psychology class, you will likely remember that experiment where a bell was rung every time a dog was to be given food. After a while, the dog would start to salivate upon hearing that bell because he knew food was coming. Well, as we age, our bladder seems conditioned to go whenever it's in proximity to a bathroom. Our brain knows why we are headed there, and our bladder picks up on that really fast. Soon, we're in a frantic race against the urge to pee. This urge can take over our entire body! If we are being open with each other, then we can probably admit to a time or two when that Pavlovian response kicked in, *ahem,* a little *too* early.

I know I can.

I remember one time when I was going to a high-profile black-tie event, and I was wearing this fabulous, long, slinky, black beaded gown. Like many formal gowns, the look required that I wear a pair of Spanx underneath to smooth any lines and, you know, keep everything where it's supposed to be. The undergarment probably cost well over a hundred dollars. I called it my *hundred-dollar torture device.* Have you ever tried to pee while wearing Spanx and a gown that extends to the floor? Do you know how hard it is to take off a Spanx undergarment while holding at least a yard of heavy beaded material up around your boobs? I can tell you, it's not easy. It actually takes two hands. And, when you've *really* gotta go, it can feel like a race to the finish line. I'll cut to the chase: That fancy pair of Spanx lost the race. Thankfully, I was not on a red carpet at the time. But even in the stall with, well, let's call it my wet scuba suit, I didn't know what to do now.

Okay, now what do I do?

I knew I couldn't stay in that bathroom stall all night. I had to make my exit and mingle back in with the crowd. I decided I had no choice. I pulled off the Spanx — yes, that really expensive undergarment — and I stuffed it into the tiny box inside the stall provided for sanitary items. I know what you're thinking. *What? Leave behind a pair of pricey Spanx?* But, come on, I had no choice! My tiny jeweled evening bag barely held my lipstick and blush; it certainly didn't have the space for a pair of soaked Spanx to fit. So I ditched the darn thing, dropped my dress back down, reapplied my lipstick, and sauntered back out into the crowd . . . commando.

As the evening went on, no matter with

whom I was having a conversation, all I could think was, *OMG, I'm here talking to so and so and I'm so bare assed.* Honestly, there were a few times when I couldn't wipe the Cheshire cat grin off my face.

As it turns out, *not quite making it to the loo in time* is a rather common problem for women as they age. Occasional leaking is a common problem, too, and not only for older women. It often happens to women who have recently delivered a child. Many new moms find that they leak when they laugh, when they pick up their baby, and definitely when they start to do sit ups and other *core work* in their mommy bootcamp class.

What many ladies do when they find this happening is to stock up on protective panty liners, or if you're like me, you just make sure you go to the bathroom more often in hopes of staying ahead of the game. Needless to say, I avoid jumping jacks and trampolines! Oh, and running too. Okay, so you already know that I'm not a big fan of running, and this is as good an excuse as any not to do it.

One of the biggest mistakes that many of us make is that we start drinking less water as a way to avoid excessive trips to the bathroom. As we discussed in the previous chapter, restricting our fluid intake can actually make the problem worse. It seems logical to drink less water; after all, doesn't less liquid translate to less peeing? It sounds like the right solution but by restricting our water intake, our urine can become more concentrated, which can irritate the bladder and, in turn, cause an increase in the frequency and the urgency to go.

If you too suffer from the same challenges, try adhering to my motto, which is, "Never pass up an opportunity to pee!"

A Lesson in Leaking

Okay, ladies, now it's time for *A Lesson in Leaking.* Stick with me here . . . there are two main types of bladder leakage: stress incontinence and urge incontinence.

Stress incontinence typically leaks a small amount of urine upon laughing, sneezing, or straining. Childbirth is a major factor in causing it, as well as having a chronic cough, obesity, or a hysterectomy. It's a mechanical issue that results from insufficient support of the bladder.

Urge incontinence, also called overactive bladder, is caused by an abnormal stimulation of nerves to the bladder. It gives us the sensation of having "to go" all the time. It can also cause the bladder to empty involuntarily and without warning.

Leaking when we cough or laugh (stress incontinence) is actually common for women. In fact, as many as one in four say they experience this. Unfortunately, some won't go for help because they believe that any kind of leaking is normal for a woman and that nothing can be done. However, there have been a lot of advances in the treatment of urinary incontinence in the past 10 years. Treatment options include behavioral therapy, medications, medical devices, and surgery. For the majority of people, it is 100 percent treatable, and most of the time a non-surgical treatment is recommended

There are medications to treat the symptoms of urinary frequency (urge incontinence) that can help prevent the uncontrollable muscle contractions leading to an overactive bladder and leaking.

A healthy bladder eliminates between 5 to 9 times a day, and typically once, or at most, twice a night. If we find ourselves waking up to pee more than that, the cause could be as simple as drinking too much fluid during the evening or we may have a condition called *nocturia*. Aging is one of the biggest factors in developing this condition. Older women produce less of the antidiuretic hormone that helps us retain fluid and decrease urine production, especially during the nighttime hours. Then, too, our bladder muscles get weaker as we age and as a result, our bladders actually hold less liquid.

There are other things that can cause us to go to the bathroom more often during the night including drinking alcohol, caffeinated beverages, and consuming products with artificial sweeteners. Alcohol and caffeinated beverages are diuretics, which cause our body to produce more urine. Other common causes are bladder infections and urinary tract infections.

If you find that you seem to always wake up to relieve yourself between 1:00 a.m. to 3:00 a.m., it may be your liver that's stirring you from your sleep. In Chinese medicine, our body's organs each have an allotted time during a 24-hour cycle when they are most actively doing their jobs, and from 1:00 a.m. to 3:00 a.m. is primetime for your liver to get to work.

You could be suffering from a fatty liver or nonalcoholic fatty liver (a condition called NAFL), especially if you eat a lot of sugar, trans fat, and processed food. A little fat is fine for your liver, but if it is overloaded with fat, it must work harder. Sugar causes insulin levels to shoot up, and this can also make the liver work extra hard trying to eliminate the excess chemicals that the sugar overload produces.

Our modern diet and lifestyle can put a lot of stress on our body, whether that stress is from eating too much refined sugar and fatty foods, consuming too much alcohol or some other stimulant, or simply having too much tension — or how about this, a combination of all of these! Yikes! This unhealthy mix can cause the liver to become toxic and overworked. The liver needs energy to do its job effectively, and it gets that energy from glycogen, aka, the body's own natural sugar stores. But herein lies the problem — our body produces adrenaline when we're stressed and the production of adrenaline also uses glycogen. When we are under pressure all day long, our adrenaline is pumping and our blood sugar levels are both rising and falling. By the time it's 1:00 a.m., there simply isn't enough glycogen left for our liver to do its job. So the body has to produce *more* adrenaline, and, of course, adrenaline is meant to keep us amped up — awake — and so it does just that. Bingo, we're wide-eyed and restless, and on top of that, we have to pee again. Ugh.

There are a number of ways to reduce stress on your liver, not the least of which includes eating regular healthy meals and avoiding caffeine, alcohol, and junk foods. This will help balance your blood sugar levels, which will help keep your adrenaline levels to a minimum, leaving enough glycogen for your liver to stay happy and productive.

The first line of treatment for most women dealing with incontinence is behavioral therapy, which includes bladder training, scheduled bathroom trips, exercises to strengthen the pelvic floor muscles, and fluid and diet management. These are what experts recommend trying first.

Hormone replacement is also now being used. There is an estrogen therapy, administered via a vaginal cream, ring, or patch, that can reduce the atrophy of the lining of the urethra and vagina in postmenopausal women. Antibiotics may be prescribed when incontinence has been caused by a urinary tract infection.

In addition, there are some medical devices that may help. A urethral insert, which is like a tampon that a woman inserts into her urethra, usually helps prevent leakage during such physical activities as tennis or jogging. This device acts as a plug to prevent leakage and is then removed to urinate. There is also an intra-vaginal device, called a pessary, which is a stiff ring that it inserted into your vagina and helps supports the bladder. It is similar to a diaphragm, however, so a doctor must place this device and it requires regular follow-up visits for it to be taken out, examined, and cleaned.

Surgery is another option, but only after all other treatment options have been tried. There are a number of surgical alternatives available. I recommend you consult with your physician to explore them together.

If you don't want to have surgery and have had no success with the medicines available, PTNS or percutaneous tibial nerve stimulation is an option. Using this technique, a doctor inserts a fine needle electrode in the nerve just above your ankle and a mild electrical impulse is delivered to the 4 nerves of the spine that control bladder function. This procedure is done in a doctor's office and involves a series of 12 treatments, each given a week apart. Improvement can be seen within the first couple of weeks.

Believe it or not, some women are turning to Botox to relieve an overactive bladder. *Whaaat? Botox? Like the stuff women use on their foreheads to smooth out wrinkles and frown lines?* Yep, the same stuff. Kind of ironic, huh? Since an overactive bladder is probably the reason you're frowning in the first place. Only, in this case, doctors inject the botulinum toxin into the bladder muscle to help it relax so that a woman has greater control over emptying her bladder. A needle is inserted using a long tube called a cysto-scope that extends up into the bladder. The effects last for about nine months. This method is only recommended if a woman's symptoms can't be controlled with behavioral therapies, medications, or a combination of both.

If you think you're suffering from an overactive bladder, here are some simple behavioral or lifestyle changes that experts recommend for relieving symptoms.

Lighten Up
Being overweight can weaken our pelvic floor muscles because of the pressure the fatty tissue puts on the bladder. Sometimes losing weight clears up the problem completely.

Stay Active
We shouldn't try to manage leakage by avoiding exercise in order to stay dry. This will simply deprive us of the vigorous activ-

ity the rest of our body needs — activity that is essential for good health. So don't give up your favorite pastimes.

Kegels to the Rescue

Kegels are the go-to exercise for strengthening the muscles supporting the bladder and uterus. If you're not sure where these muscles are, simply imagine that you are peeing and picture yourself trying to stop the flow of urine. The muscles you use when attempting to hold back the flow are the muscles we're looking to strengthen.

Now for the exercise: Tighten and pull up the pelvic floor muscles and hold the squeeze for as long as you can, then relax those muscles. Every time you do this exercise, try to hold each squeeze for a little longer (up to 10 seconds) and relax for 3 or 4 seconds before starting again. Don't expect overnight results; it can take a few months before you see improvement, but it's worth the wait for quality of life.

I have a confession. I always hated doing Kegels. I found them so darn annoying that I never used to do them. My internist told me what she tells all of her female patients: Just remember to do 10 Kegels every time you stop at a red light. Try it. It works. And tell me you don't smile when you look at the person in the car next to you. They have no idea that you're in the middle of doing a workout *down there*! I've got to admit, ever since she gave me the idea, I go into action at every red light. If you ever pull up next to me, well, now you know what I'm up to! Thanks, Dr. Lithgow!

Protect Your Core

I was surprised when I first heard that the pelvic floor was considered part of the core. Understanding that encourages us to choose activities that are pelvic-floor friendly, such as Pilates, and avoid those that are not, such as crunches, which may be good for a six-pack but I've been warned can sometimes worsen this situation.

Avoid High Impact Exercise

High impact exercise can put a lot of pressure on our pelvic floor muscles so jogging and aerobics might not be the right exercise to choose.

Avoid Lifting

Lifting can strain the pelvic floor muscles, so avoid it if possible. When we need to lift something, like our grandchildren, pets, or heavy bags from the grocery store, it is recommended that we use our legs and tighten our pelvic floor muscle before and during lifting.

Eat the Right Foods

Foods that are spicy and acidic, such as citrus fruits and juices, can irritate the bladder. Too much sugar and refined carbohydrates can also have an adverse effect because they upset our blood glucose levels. It's best to think *fresh* and focus on getting plenty of veggies, fruits, and lean protein when buying groceries. The thing to remember is that if we stress out and produce lots of adrenaline all day long and make poor food choices as well, we're likely to be awake between 1:00 to 3:00 in the morning.

Drink Plenty of Water

I know it seems counterintuitive, but as discussed, drinking six to eight glasses of water a day really is important. A lot of people who suffer from urinary incontinence avoid drinking fluids, which only makes incontinence worse and can also result in constipation. So without enough water in your system you may find yourself racing for the bathroom or staying in there way too long. Either way, it's nothing you want to explain at a dinner party.

242

Avoid Caffeine

Drinks such as coffee and soda are a no-no. They can irritate the bladder and make incontinence worse. Caffeine is a diuretic that results in rapid filling of the bladder and a powerful urge to urinate, even when the bladder is not full. Remember that many teas, energy drinks, and even hot chocolate contain caffeine. Carbonated drinks and the artificial sweetener aspartame can also cause urgency. If you must have your stimulant fix, at least avoid consuming caffeine and sugar after 3:00 p.m.

Avoid Alcohol

Alcohol is also a diuretic, so it makes a person urinate more often. I understand that having urgency issues can *drive one to drink* as the saying goes, but remember the reverse is actually true.

Quit Smoking

Anyone who smokes is putting themselves at risk of incontinence because coughing puts undue strain on the pelvic floor muscles.

Develop Good Toilet Habits

Yes, we are going to talk about *potty training for the aging.* So here we go. Wait until your bladder is full to urinate and never delay the urge to empty your bowels. Don't rush it — straining to empty your bowels weakens your pelvic floor muscles. If you suffer from constipation, increase your fiber intake and exercise more. There is evidence that changing the way you sit and use your muscles can help to empty your bowels as well. Thus, the Squatty Potty was born — and it works. This tiny stool helps you to sit comfortably on the commode with your knees raised above your hips the way they would be if you were actually squatting. Squatting is the way we moved our bowels long before modern conveniences came into being. The position relaxes the puborectalis muscle so you can empty your bowels safely and completely. Just ask your dogs; it works well for them. Quite often nature has the answers.

Power Down at Bedtime

You might be asking what the use of our technology at night has to do with incontinence. Well, reducing technology at bedtime can help lessen stress, which will help keep our adrenaline levels to a minimum. So here is one more reason to turn off your phone, computer, iPad, and TV at least one hour before retiring to bed. Use this time to unwind and relax.

Protect Yourself with Panty Liners

I know this is something women don't always want to discuss, but we've all seen the commercials, and the fact is, pads work well. Recognizing what a common problem this is for women, companies who make feminine products are even designing protective underwear that is pretty, and, I dare say in some cases, even sexy looking. Just google "incontinence underwear for women."

With that, I have to share a story with you that frankly almost made me pee my pants. I was on vacation with my family when I got a call from my agent asking if I'd be interested in doing a TV commercial for a popular line of disposable absorbent panties. I was so amused by the offer that I had to share it with everyone present. My teenagers immediately said that if I was ever in one of those commercials, they'd never be able to show their faces in school again. We all started to giggle . . . and, well, you know the rest of the story.

Gotta run. Nature is calling!

CHAPTER 15
SLEEPING BEAUTY WAS
ON TO SOMETHING

"Going to bed early.
Not leaving the house.
Not going to a party.
My childhood punishments have become
my adult goals."
— A PINTEREST PAL

Please don't let any prince kiss me — I need
my rest!

Sleeping Beauty was not just a pretty face.
She was the poster child for excellent self-
care! Her story reveals an anti-aging practice
we should all try more often. This might be
why the old hag of a witch hated her so.
Experts say that *sleep* is the secret ingredi-
ent not only to good health and a clear,
focused mind, but it's also one of the best
magic potions for beautiful looking skin,
like Sleeping Beauty's.

I know that when I have a sleepless night,
I not only feel physically tired and less

246

focused, I'm also more likely to see fine lines on my face and to have a dull, blotchy complexion the next morning. I feel like a sleepless night leaves us looking like we're hungover and certainly less healthy. Researchers concur. They say we *are* less healthy when we don't get enough zzzz's. Ugh!

When you get me started on the topic of sleep, or the lack thereof, you've hit a nerve. Sleep has always been my nemesis. I've just never been good at getting enough.

I've always yearned for more of it. I've been struggling with this issue my entire adult life. Not only did I get up every day for twenty years at 3:30 a.m. to appear on *Good Morning America,* but the demands of being a mom to seven children meant there never seemed to be enough hours in my day for sleep!

I'm insanely jealous of how long my teen-aged kids can snooze! Often when they are whiling the day away in bed, my husband and I want to go into their rooms to check their pulses just to make sure they're still alive! Is there something wrong with them that they can sleep that long? The truth is, it's not uncommon for teens to sleep like that. I think we only react the way we do because we secretly covet their rest!

Rest and Sleep Are Essential for Our Brains to Renew!

There is a tremendous amount of research on the effects sleep has on our health. Many major league sports teams employ sleep coaches to work with their players so they can perform at their maximum level at game time. A lot of professional teams contractually require their players to get 10 hours of sleep a night during their season. But what about the rest of us mortal humans? Health experts say adults need between seven to nine hours of sleep every night. *Really? Do they mean like every single night?* Oh boy, I'm in trouble.

According to the Centers for Disease Control and Prevention, an estimated 50 to 70 million adults in this country have a sleep or wakefulness disorder, which can wreak havoc on our health. While we are sound asleep, our body is hard at work, making repairs like a crew of construction workers toiling away on the night shift. When we are in deep sleep, our human growth hormone production increases. The normal release of this hormone plays a key role in healing cells and tissues throughout our body, including our skin. Good sleep improves our heart health and can lower inflammation, which also wards off wrinkles and leads to a clearer countenance. Getting an adequate amount of sleep can help us maintain a healthy weight too.

Do Our Sleep Needs Change as We Age?

One of the challenges to healthy aging is ensuring that we are getting enough sleep and rest. There is a myth that older people require less sleep, but experts have told me that is really not true. *All* adults, regardless of age, should have the requisite hours of sleep each night.

Just because it might be *difficult* to get a good night's sleep, doesn't mean we don't *need* it. For a number of reasons, older people often have trouble falling *and* staying asleep. A lot of us find that we wake up three or four times a night. This could be because our sleep is less deep and therefore not as restful. Also, for a lot of people, sleep is interrupted by frequent trips to the bathroom. *Sometimes I feel like I'm just at an age where an* all-nighter *means that I didn't sleep a wink because I was up to pee so often!*

All joking aside, why is it that older adults sleep less? The answer is that our body changes as we age, and these changes can impact the length and quality of our sleep. For instance, we secrete less of two important sleep hormones: melatonin and growth hormone.

You've probably heard of melatonin and that's for a good reason. The amount of this hormone we have in our body dictates the *length and timing* of our sleep cycle. As our melatonin levels decline, many older adults feel sleepy in the early evening and they wake up practically at dawn the next morning. They may also have more trouble falling asleep. When this growth hormone is present in the right amounts, it can positively influence *the quality* of our sleep. It is what makes children slumber so deeply. As we age and our body secretes less and less of this hormone, achieving that same kind of sound, cellular-building sleep we had in our youth becomes more difficult.

Melatonin also works with another hormone called cortisol for a different purpose. Together they prepare us for the two opposite ends of the sleep-wake cycle. Cortisol is a stress hormone that typically kick-starts our day. It is usually secreted just before we wake up in the morning so we feel refreshed and energized for the tasks ahead of us. Melatonin, on the other hand, is produced in the evening as natural light fades, helping us to feel relaxed and sleepy in anticipation of bedtime.

If we are prone to anxiety and chronic

stress, our body produces more cortisol. If excess cortisol remains in our system for an extended period of time, it can overwhelm our liver and wreak havoc with our sleep patterns. When there is too much cortisol in the system due to stress, the balance between cortisol (which wakes us up) and melatonin (which winds us down) is upset. Basically, too much stress leads to too much cortisol, which leads to an inability to sleep (aka insomnia). Now remember, the liver is on the clock doing its job between the hours of 1:00 a.m. to 3:00 a.m. If we are awake at that time, flooded with cortisol, and flooded with adrenaline (another byproduct of stress) the liver has a big problem. In order to do its work well, it needs energy. It gets that energy from glycogen, which it takes from our body's natural sugar supply. The problem is that adrenaline production also uses glycogen. So now because we've been stressed all day, there's no glycogen for the liver when it needs it! Ponder that while you're sitting up in bed. Is it any wonder we look like crap the next morning?

Of course, menopause and other health conditions, such as arthritis pain and diabetes, can also have a negative effect on our sleep. Menopause, for instance, can result in night sweats and other symptoms that keep us up at night.

So how dangerous is it not to get a decent amount of sleep? It's bad. Lack of sleep is tied to myriad health problems including obesity and high blood pressure, not to mention daytime sleepiness, which can lead to loss of productivity, traffic accidents, job-related accidents, and more.

But instead of getting stressed out about all of this and losing even more sleep, I did some research, and came up with a list of suggested ways we could all get a better night's rest.

TO HELP GET A GOOD NIGHT'S SLEEP

1. Have a Bedtime Ritual

As parents, we have all been told to create a nightly ritual for our children so that they can naturally transition into a sleepy state. Well, the prescription is the same for adults. It is advised that we start our ritual about 30 minutes before we slip into bed so we can help release any stressful thoughts from earlier in the day and be ready to go to sleep once we tuck in.

For those of us who have a tough time turning our mind off at night, experts suggest that we take a warm bath, write in a journal, listen to soft music, or meditate using an app so we can bring closure to our day. I can't tell you that I've ever taken a warm bath right before bed to get myself to sleep, nor do I journal at night because it tends to stimulate my mind. I prefer doing that during the day when it won't cause me to lie awake *thinking* about everything I just wrote.

Instead of what the experts advise, my husband and I usually retreat to the bedroom when primetime TV shows air. I know, we are *so* old school. We tend to watch shows at their regularly scheduled times. The word "binge" is still associated with eating for us, not with watching TV. Don't laugh; we already get enough teasing from our children for viewing television like such old fogies.

Candidly, there were so many years when I couldn't stay up to watch primetime because I needed to be at the studio before dawn the next morning for hair and make-up. Seriously, I had to be camera-ready and well versed on any breaking news before the rest of you were even awake. Now, watching nighttime TV is my guilty pleasure.

253

But don't do as I do. Do as the experts tell you to. Sleep authorities all warn that watching that blue backlit screen of our TVs, computers, and phones at night can stimulate our brain and wreak havoc with our sleep. I keep promising myself that I'll turn the TV off and go to bed earlier, but admittedly this is one of my weaknesses. Hopefully you will be better disciplined — and better rested — than me!

Most sleep experts also warn against reading in bed. They say this too stimulates the mind and encourages wakefulness. I have friends who swear that a little quiet reading never fails to make them sleepy, but I'm with the experts on this one. Whenever I take a book to bed, it's a total disaster. I suppose if the ones I chose weren't such page-turners it would be okay. But I get so caught up in the story that I keep convincing myself to read just one more chapter. As proof that the sleep researchers are right, I'm always groggy the next day!

2. Meditation Apps Are the New-Age Version of Counting Sheep

One of my favorite ways to nod off is listening to a meditation app that uses *progressive muscle relaxation.* I've taught my kids to do this type of exercise on their own, without the app. Try it; I think you'll like it. Start by concentrating on your toes, first tensing all the muscles as tightly as you can, and then completely relaxing them. Now move your attention up to your ankles and so on, working your way body part by body part from your feet up to the top of your head. When I took a trip and shared a bed with my younger girls, we did this exercise together and compared notes the next morning about who got to sleep the fastest. My daughter exclaimed, "I only made it to my knees, Mom!"

If you find that every time you close your eyes and try to think of nothing, your entire to-do list comes rushing to mind, don't worry; you are not alone. It happens to me too. Trying one of the many guided mediation apps that are available online and in the app store can help. I especially like Headspace and Calm.

3. Take a Hot Bath
If falling asleep is a challenge for you, experts suggest that a hot bath might help. Bear with me, as this is tricky. Studies have shown that a colder core body tem-

perature can help induce sleep, which is why some scientists recommend going to bed in a cold room. At night our body temperature naturally drops, which is what signals the production of melatonin, the sleep hormone. When we soak in a hot bath, our body temperature rises, but when we get out of the tub, our body rapidly cools down, bringing on the production of melatonin. Get it? The sudden drop in body temperature after we get out of a warm bath triggers melatonin to get us drowsy. That bath has actually prepared us for sleep. I can't say that I've done this before, but hey, it's worth a try.

4. Wake Up and Go to Bed at the Same Time Each Day
Going to bed and waking up at the same time every day is highly recommended since it trains our body to sleep on a schedule. If we can maintain a schedule for several weeks, the experts say we will probably fall asleep easier and faster. And we'll likely feel more refreshed upon waking.

Needless to say, sleep was often a topic of conversation around the GMA studio since we all needed it, wanted it, dreamed of it — or should I say *daydreamed* about it? I remember interviewing a sleep expert on *Good Morning America* once who told Charlie Gibson and me that we should stay on our weekday early morning schedule right through the weekend. I looked at him in horror and asked, "Are you telling us not to stay up late or sleep in on weekends?" You've got to be kidding me? That's not happening!

The sleep expert went on to tell us that our body adjusts to changes in our sleep schedule at a rate of one hour per day. What he was saying was that if one wakes up at 6:30 a.m. on weekdays, but at 8:30 a.m. on weekends, that's a two-hour difference and therefore we would need two days to adjust. He was basically telling us that even with our crazy schedules, if we slept late on the weekends, we probably wouldn't be sleeping well again until Wednesday of each week. *Really?* I'm not here to dispute the experts, but as you can imagine, Charlie and I never took that advice to heart. We often discussed our sleep patterns, or lack thereof, with each other. Charlie's problem was late night sports on TV; he just couldn't turn off a good game. For me, the sleep challenges evolved with my kids. In the early days on GMA my daughters were babies and by the time I left they were teenagers. But do I really need to explain why I never got enough sleep? It seems to me as if the answer is obvious to every working mother!

5. Exercise Daily

According to the experts, a daily exercise habit is one of the best ways to improve our chances of falling asleep quickly and to remain sleeping deeply. Exercise, particularly during the morning or afternoon, can affect our sleep quality by raising our body temperature a few degrees. Then later in the evening, when our internal thermostat drops back to a normal range, this can trigger feelings of drowsiness and help us drop off to sleep.

Sleep experts recommend that we never exercise within three hours of bedtime, because this can stimulate our endorphins and not allow enough time for that rise and fall in body temperature to occur, making it difficult to fall asleep. That works for me. I don't know about you, but I'm usually too tired to think about working out right before I go to bed.

6. Get Some Sunlight

I thrive on sunlight — it makes me happy and gives me energy. Sleep experts say that spending time outdoors in the sun also helps to regulate our circadian clock. The contrast between being outdoors in the daylight and being indoors as the evening grows dark signals to our body when it's time to produce melatonin, the hormone that regulates our sleep cycle.

The reason why we feel energized and drowsy around the same times every day is because we fall into a circadian rhythm. This rhythm is like a 24-hour internal clock running in the background of our brain. It cycles between sleepiness and alertness at regular intervals. When we stay true to that clock, we create a rhythm that tells our body when it's time to wake and when it's time to rest.

I take melatonin every night to help signal when it's time to sleep and I swear by it! Experts also recommend at least two hours of exposure to bright light each day. The morning sunlight is especially helpful as that is when cortisol, the hormone that rouses us, typically kicks in. So rather than stay snuggled in our darkened cocoon, we should open up our drapes or blinds each day and let the morning sunshine in.

7. Make Your Bedroom Dark When You Sleep

The contrast between light during the day and dark at night helps to reinforce our bodies' natural rhythms. My husband and I close our blinds every night before we climb into bed to help reduce the light in the room. But when I began to look into the connection between darkness and getting a truly good night's sleep, I found that shutting the blinds was only a start.

Our bodies are programmed to get sleepy when it gets dark. If our eyes sense darkness, our hypothalamus will tell our body to release melatonin, which, as you know, helps us to fall asleep easily. If there's too much light in the room, our brains won't receive the correct signals and falling asleep might be delayed. By the way, light actually inhibits the secretion of melatonin.

In order to ease into nighttime, it's recommended that we dim the lights as we're getting ready for bed. That means we should turn off any bright overhead lights and turn on a soft bedside lamp. If we have a digital clock or any other glowing electronics on that nightstand, it's advised we turn it around so that it's hidden from our view. Even a nightlight in our bedroom can disturb melatonin production. So put that night light in the hall or in the bathroom — just in case Mother Nature calls — and don't flip on a ceiling light if you get up in the middle of the night. That can really affect your melatonin levels. Even a streetlamp or bright moonlight coming through the window can interfere with your sleep.

Why is melatonin so important? When our body doesn't produce enough, it not only impacts our ability to get to sleep and to stay asleep, it also impacts our hormone function and has even been connected to depression and an increased risk of cancer.

8. Cut Down on Catnaps

I don't know about you, but I've never been able to sneak in a catnap during the day. I remember Charlie Gibson used to be able to go to sleep for 10 to 15 minutes right on the set with everything going on around him. How the heck did he do that? I always teased him about it, but quite honestly, I was totally jealous. People swear that taking naps refreshes them and makes them more productive, and many experts agree. However, while napping can be great (or so they tell me), if you are napping more than 20 minutes a day or too late in the day, it may be interfering with your sleep at night.

9. Avoid Caffeine, Alcohol, and Nicotine My husband can drink a cup of strong black coffee after dinner and still fall sound asleep minutes after his head hits the pillow. (That's a man for you. Annoying, isn't it?) I limit my caffeine to a morning cup. If you are one of those people who are caffeine sensitive, then avoid drinking coffee, tea, or any other caffeinated beverages up to six hours before bedtime.

An evening drink of alcohol can also impact our sleep. We might nod off just fine, but we will likely wake up in the middle of the night. Even a small glass of wine can make it more difficult to stay asleep. This is caused by a rebound in blood sugar and a withdrawal from the alcohol after it is metabolized.

For every drink we have, we need to give our body at least an hour to process it before trying to fall asleep. Or just avoid alcohol after dinner-time in order to sleep more soundly. Nicotine is also a stimulant that can keep a person awake. And that's the least of the trouble that nicotine will cause.

10. Check Your Meds

As we age, it is also more likely that we are taking one or more medications. Many medications can interfere with our sleep. If you think this might be an issue for you, ask your doctor to change your prescription to something that doesn't cause you to lose sleep. If that is not possible, check to see if you can change the time of day you take that medication as the further away from bedtime you take it, the better off you are.

11. Only Sleep and Have Sex in the Bedroom

Sleep experts say the bedroom should be used only for sleep and sex. *Wait, that means no reading in bed? And no watching TV there either?* Well, no wonder I'm having trouble going to sleep! According to the experts, watching TV and reading can confuse our body into thinking that we are still in the active hours of our day, mak-

ing it difficult to fall asleep. Okay, I can attest to that one.

Instead, sleep experts recommend that we
give ourselves fifteen minutes to fall
asleep. If we haven't dozed off by then,
we should get out of bed and do *something
boring.* Seriously, I'm not kidding. We
aren't supposed to do anything that will
stimulate us. That means no TV screens,
no computer screens, nothing that is
backlit. The only stimulation before sleep
should be sex.

Sex, on the other hand, not only helps us
sleep but it will also help us live longer by
relieving stress and releasing feel-good
hormones like oxytocin. Experts say that
having satisfying sex two to three times
per week can add as many as three years
to our life. Regular sex lowers blood pressure, improves sleep, boosts immunity,
and protects our heart. Having sex can
also burn an impressive number of calories
— sometimes as many as the equivalent
of running for 30 minutes. *Wow.* Which
would you prefer? For those of you reading who are not married or in a relationship, you can do this alone and then fall
right to sleep without even having to

cuddle (most menopausal women can't handle too much contact at bedtime as men give off a lot of body heat typically).

One thing I know for sure is that when I do get a restful night of sleep and I wake up naturally, which means without the help of an alarm clock or a dog jumping on the bed and licking my face, I feel like a million bucks. Seriously, I smile even before I open my eyes because I can literally *feel* the healthy effects of deep sleep. I also know that I won't have to rely on coffee and/or concealer to send me off for the day. Frown lines? Gone. Blotchy skin? Gone. Sparkle in the eyes? Present and radiant! Spring in my step? Oh yeah!

The best news in all of this is that the world's greatest natural beauty treatment is free of charge. *It's sleep!*

CHAPTER 16
DID YOU KNOW
CHOCOLATE MAKES YOUR
CLOTHES SHRINK?

"Chocolate comes from cocoa, which is a
tree. That makes it a plant . . . so
chocolate is a salad."
— UNKNOWN

I'm confused . . . is chocolate on the no-no
list? Yes, traditionally it's been an indulgent
dessert, but these days I see dark chocolate
on almost every list of superfoods! The way
I look at, that means dark chocolate *must*
slow down the aging process. Come on,
maybe it's not true, but do we dare take
that chance?

"If we're not meant to have midnight
snacks, why is there a light in the fridge?"
— UNKNOWN

Recently I finished eating dinner with my
family and experienced that weird uncomfortable phenomenon of still being hungry.
How could that be? It didn't make any

sense. But there it was for me to deal with.

I tried very discreetly, so that my family wouldn't notice, to toast a whole wheat English muffin and add some raspberry jam. I justified it by telling myself that it was my dessert. Wait. Better yet, I thought, this is actually a health food; a serving of whole grains, and a serving of fruit. Yeah. That's what it is. I thoroughly entertained myself with that rationale. I actually laughed out loud and suddenly . . . my husband and kids looked up at me in sync and saw that I was eating something more after we had all just finished having dinner.

Busted!

If we indulge too often and find ourselves carrying around extra pounds, it can take a significant toll on our health. It increases the risk of Type 2 diabetes, heart disease, stroke, many types of cancer, sleep apnea, and other debilitating and chronic illnesses.

Processed foods, frozen dinners, and drive-thru meals have provided us with a tremendous amount of convenience in this modern world, but if we want to know how to eat more wisely to ensure our health, we must look to countries where they prepare and eat fresh foods on a daily basis.

In his fascinating book *The Blue Zones,* author Dan Buettner identifies pockets in the world where people live exponentially longer than the rest of us. He attributes their healthier states and increased longevity to their lifestyles.

From Sardinia to a place a little closer to home, Loma Linda, California, (where the life expectancy is 10 years longer than the national average!) residents of these blue zones are said not only to eat fresh, locally grown or homegrown foods in most instances, but they walk everywhere, laugh with friends often, value and prioritize their family, and celebrate their elders too. That lifestyle means they enjoy a higher nutrition level, a lower stress level, and a greater degree of happiness, which obviously add up to a longer life span.

All of these cultures drink lots of water, others enjoy antioxidant-rich herbal teas, and some shy away from smoking, drinking coffee, and alcoholic beverages. While they all exercise daily and generally keep an active social life, they include naps or other forms of relaxation into their day too. Interestingly, residents of one area said they purposefully do not hurry through life. Can't you just feel your tensions melting away?

Many residents of these blue zones get lots of sunshine just by virtue of their location, and others make a point of bringing light into their life by attending religious services and/or by having a sense of purpose and community. A deep spiritual life of one kind or another seems to be an important factor to maintaining a far less stressed general population.

Upon examining life in these sun-filled havens, we find that the people who live there aren't eating processed or fat-laden fast foods; they aren't drinking sugary sodas; and they tend to build an equal amount of vigorous activity and rest into their daily lives. That sure seems to be a recipe for youth.

It also should be noted that these cultures eat food in reasonable quantities and enjoy their meals in one another's company.

Buettner's study also looked at the oldest Japanese people and found that they tend to stop eating when they are feeling only about 80 percent full.

Researchers at St. Louis University confirmed Buettner's findings that eating less helps us age at a slower pace. Their study found that limiting calories lowered the production of T3, which is a thyroid hormone that decelerates metabolism and speeds up the aging process.

So how do we start eating less on a regular

basis? While I'm not a nutritionist, I've learned over the years that it's very important to eat heart-healthy foods. I've tried countless diets. Some worked . . . kind of. But I'd often gain the weight back after I reached my goal. What I have found successful, however, is following an eating plan. You know, these are programs that are not really diets so much as ways to incorporate healthy foods into our life on a long-term basis. When I was on my chemo regimen I worked with a nutritionist, Dr. Rob Zembroski, the author of *Rebuild,* who had me follow a no sugar, no wheat, no dairy plan. The first time he told me about it I said, "What's left to eat?" He knew right then that he had his work cut out for him. But as it happened, I learned quickly that I could enjoy tasty, satisfying meals featuring nutrient-dense proteins such as grilled chicken or seafood, along with lots and lots of vegetables. I could also eat carbohydrates such as sweet potatoes, quinoa, couscous, and brown rice. I just had to say no to white potatoes and white rice. Fruits were included, but not too much at one time for me, since they can raise your blood sugar level, which we were careful not to do while I was being treated. I will tell you that I had very few of the yucky side effects that cancer patients usually complain about. And I certainly didn't protest when I lost a good percentage of my body fat!

More recently, I've had tremendous success following what I learned in *The Stark Naked 21-Day Metabolic Reset* by nutrition and fitness expert Brad Davidson. (By the way, my good friend Laura also worked with Brad on his book.) After having so much aggressive chemo, and also from just plain aging, my liver wasn't functioning properly; I could tell that I was storing fat around my waist. That scared me. I know how dangerous that is for our health. So I went on Brad's 21-day plan and it solved all of my digestive issues. I also lost 12 pounds and almost two inches around my middle. And that's not all; I'd had chronic pain in my hip joints and within a week all that pain was gone. Apparently, this way of eating reduced the inflammation in my body. On this plan, I start my day with a warm glass of water, made all the more refreshing by including half a lemon. I drink a green smoothie every morning, too, blending water and ice with spinach, celery, berries, watermelon, and avocado. What doesn't taste better with a little avocado? I tried a lot of the other smoothie recipes in the book and benefited from the variety. I never really missed my eggs, bacon, and toast. Well, maybe I did, but to me the results were so worth it. Now, as my general rule in life, I follow a combination of the Stark Naked 21-day Metabolic Reset and the Mediterranean diet, always choosing fresh foods and piling on the veggies. Thankfully, I'm not much of a dessert person, so keeping the sugar out of my diet hasn't been as difficult for me as it is for some others. Instead, I'm doomed to crave salty/crunchy foods. I just have to give in and eat some Tostitos and guacamole every now and then.

Again, I'm not a nutritionist, but I can tell you that eating clean has been best for me. Replacing fried foods and processed foods with simple nutrient-dense proteins and lots of veggies and staying away from sugar has made a huge difference in my life. To get you started, here are what nutritionists say are the basic guidelines that we should all be following.

1. **Limit saturated fats and dietary cholesterol.** These are found primarily in red meat and full-fat dairy products and can raise our total cholesterol levels.
2. **Eliminate trans fats.** These are sometimes listed on food labels as

partially hydrogenated vegetable oil, and are often used in margarines and store-bought cookies, crackers, and cakes. Trans fats raise cholesterol levels too.

3. **Eat more fiber-rich foods.** In fact, soluble fiber from foods such as beans, oats, barley, Brussels sprouts, apples, and pears are especially good for you.

4. **Choose foods rich in omega-3 fatty acids.** These include foods such as salmon, mackerel, herring, walnuts, and flaxseeds. All have many heart-healthy benefits, not the least of which is reduced blood pressure.

5. **Choose protein-rich plant foods.** You will find legumes or beans, nuts, and seeds in this category.

6. **Keep your plate colorful with fruits and vegetables.** Vibrant, richly colored fruits and vegetables are nutritional powerhouses filled with vitamins and fiber that can lower our risks for myriad diseases. A plant-based diet will help keep us healthy and extend our lives.

"Food is the most abused anxiety drug. Exercise is the most underutilized antidepressant."
— BILL PHILLIPS; AUTHOR OF
BODY FOR LIFE

Obesity is a national crisis and has been one of the biggest contributors in driving up our health care spending over the past 20 years. The U.S. is literally *saturated* with fast-food restaurants; our supermarkets have aisles and aisles of junk food; and, of course, technologies have rendered much of the population sedentary.

An alarming forecast regarding obesity in America has had health experts fearing a dramatic jump in health care costs if nothing is done to bring rising weights under control. The study, first conducted in 2012, warned that 42 percent of Americans could end up obese by 2030, and 11 percent could be severely obese (roughly 100 or more pounds over a healthy weight). This increase would mean 32 million more obese people within two decades.

We certainly have a fast food epidemic in this country! In these crazy busy lives we lead, I understand the temptation to make a quick and easy meal choice but turning to fast food regularly is a habit that can eventually become deadly. Large high-fat meals can have a variety of immediate adverse effects, which are most concerning if we already have heart disease or risk factors for it.

Super-sized meals are a super-dangerous lifestyle choice that has had a devastating effect on Americans. As obesity rates rise, experts at the Centers for Disease Control are now forecasting that this next generation may be the first generation to die before their parents. We can't let that happen.

Here's what you can take home with you after consuming just one fast food meal:

Stiffer Arteries and Reduced Blood Flow: Large high-fat meals can impair the ability of blood vessels to dilate or expand when necessary. This helps explain why people who have cardiovascular disease and who eat a large, high-fat meal, and then exercise, can get angina or even suffer a heart attack. Digesting any kind of large meal also causes our heart rate to speed up because of the increased demands from the digestive tract.

Higher Blood Pressure: A super-sized meal can trigger the release of norepinephrine, a stress hormone that can raise blood pressure and heart rate.

High Triglycerides: Any meal will raise levels of these fats in the blood, but a large meal, especially one super rich in fat or refined carbohydrates, will cause those levels to rise the most, and remain elevated for six to twelve hours. Accompany that food with any kind of alcohol, and your triglycerides will rise even higher.

Blood Sugar: If a person has diabetes, a super-sized meal can impair their body's ability to process glucose.

Heartburn: If a person is prone to heartburn, the larger the meal, the more gastric reflux they're likely to experience.

If we are a healthy person, overindulging occasionally in fast food shouldn't be a big problem. But if we have undesirable cholesterol levels, high blood pressure, diabetes, or a preexisting heart disease — or if we are already overweight or smoke — then super-sized meals can be a super-bad choice.

Here are some no-nonsense ideas that can help us become more conscious of the food choices we are making and the amount of food we are consuming.

Keep a Food Journal: I have to begin with this one since nutritionists always start clients with a journal. It helps us to become more aware of our eating habits and to take ownership of them. The first time I worked with a nutritionist, she had me keep track of everything I ate, when I ate it, where I ate it, even what I was thinking about when I ate it. Reading through that journal was a shocker. I was taken aback, and frankly embarrassed, at how much and how often I was eating. It also became apparent *why* I was sometimes eating. Can you say *boredom?* That was it, basically. I wasn't hungry. More likely, I was thirsty. What a revelation it was.

By the way, I burned that first food journal, lest anyone ever see it. If you've never done this exercise, I recommend you try it. Get a little notebook and keep it with you. After a while, just the mere fact that I had to record my food intake made me rethink whether or not I really wanted that bite of a cookie when just passing through the kitchen. If it wasn't worth the effort to write it down, it wasn't worth eating.

Limit Dinners Out: We have more control over the quantity that we eat when we cook at home. But the reason is more important than that. Restaurants are generally more interested in making their food taste better than they are interested in our health. While more restaurants today are including caloric information, they are likely using more salt and butter than we do when we cook at home. (Except for my mom; it just wasn't dinner unless the meal was laden with butter and gravy of some sort!)

Plate Your Meals: I have a big family with four teenagers who can eat me out of house and home. My kids like me to put platters of food on the table so they can choose what they want and how much they want. For me, this is a disaster, because it means that my willpower to exercise portion control is being tested at every meal. I've been trying to institute a new way of serving my family dinner: I've been *plating* meals just like they're served in a restaurant. When I do this, we have exactly the type and amount of food that is healthy (herein lies their objection), and we will then only eat what I knowingly put on our plates — no more extra helpings from the communal platters!

Eat Breakfast: I've never had trouble with this one since I tend to wake up hungry. However, my teenagers constantly run out of the house without eating a proper meal to start their day. It makes me crazy. It's been proven that we will be more alert and focused and have a better energy level if we eat a nutritious breakfast every morning.

Eat Slowly: I am embarrassed to admit that I am a fast eater. I hate it when I take the last bite of food on my plate only to look up and see that everyone else at the table is only half finished. I try to be more aware; I've even resorted to using my grandkids' tiny spoons. The reason why we want to eat slowly is that it takes about twenty minutes for our body to signal our brain that we're full. The thought of how many extra calories I consume between the timer going off in my belly and going off in my brain is enough to convince me that I need to give eating slowly a try!

Beware of Kitchen Clean-Up: Can we all just admit what sometimes happens when we're cleaning up after dinner? (Not that *I* ever nibbled on someone else's leftover pizza crust.) For those cooking the family feast and cleaning up afterward, it can really be challenging to resist one last crumb. And moms have the added temptation of dealing with the morsels left on the plates of their kids' meals! Come on. You've never indulged in a bite of that last, lonely chicken finger?

I used to work with a fitness trainer who once told me that she had a client who kept a spray can of insect killer in the kitchen. As she cleared everyone's plates from the table, she immediately doused them with the repellant. Apparently, this client had no self-control, and it was the only way to ensure that she wouldn't eat what remained on the plates. Wow, that's a bit drastic, don't you think? I'm not RAIDing her refrigerator anytime soon.

Watch Fewer Than 10 Hours of TV a Week: Do you graze while watching TV? Fortunately, I don't have too much to confess on this front, although I do like freshly popped popcorn with a good movie. Studies have shown that when we are distracted or simply not paying attention to what we're eating, we tend to eat more. A report published in the *American Journal of Clinical Nutrition* found that researchers from the University of Birmingham in the United Kingdom looked at how attention and memory affect food intake. They concluded that if we aren't mindful of what's going into our mouths, we don't process that information. That means there's no record of it in our memory bank. And without a memory of having eaten, we are more likely to eat again sooner than we might have if we ate mindfully.

Mindfulness, in the context of eating, includes noticing the colors, aromas, flavors, and textures of our food. It also means not watching television, reading a book, or working on our computer while eating.

If this is one of your weak points, then find some healthy snacks such as celery and carrots or limit your TV viewing. We all tend to have times when we snack, and we need to identify those times and prepare for them.

Leave Something on the Plate: My husband and I often go out to dinner with his parents, Janey and Donny (I'm lucky in that I have awesome in-laws), and I noticed recently that Janey rarely eats her full meal. I asked her about it, and she told me that she'd read an article that said if you left four or five bites uneaten at each meal, you could lose 9 1/2 pounds by the end of the year. She went on to say that she'd been following this plan for several months, asking the waiter to wrap up half of her dinner to go and then eating only the remaining half. She said that now she always has yummy leftovers, plus she was down five pounds.

So I did a little research and came across a book by Michael Pollan called *Food Rules: An Eater's Manual.* I was excited to find that one of Pollan's guidelines was, in fact, to *leave something on the plate.* He went on to explain that this was challenging for many people since they grew up hearing, "You can't leave the table or have dessert until you clean your plate." Many of these same people were also asked, "Do you realize how many starving children there are in this world?" Of course, the underlying message was that we were incredibly fortunate to have all this food and how wasteful it would be to leave uneaten bites on your plate. Pollan encourages readers to take this form of self-discipline and use it instead to stop eating when we're full and not when the plate is clean.

I've been working hard at following this approach to eating and I am here to tell you that while it may sound simple, it can be rather difficult. First of all, I'd start a meal with the best of intentions and before I knew it, I had inhaled every last forkful. Then, too, I found that I had a psychological reaction to looking at and scraping the uneaten food on my plate into the trash. It seemed so unnatural, and of course, wasteful. However, it made me aware of how much we are unconsciously influenced by our learned behaviors.

"The secret to living well and longer is:
Eat half, walk double,
laugh triple and love without measure."
— TIBETAN PROVERB

Walk It Off: I personally feel better when I take a walk after a meal. We've all heard that weight control is about the number of calories we take in versus the energy we expend burning those calories. But I've always felt that walks can provide so much more than just a calorie burn. They tend to ground me — to bring my senses back to what's happening around me. Taking a walk can also make me more attuned to what my body is feeling. Satisfyingly full? Or stuffed perhaps? It's good to be cognizant of how our body is experiencing a consumed meal. Sometimes I find it a helpful reminder not to overeat next time.

On that note, I want to leave you with some indelible advice offered to me by my fitness trainer, Beth. She once told me after a challenging workout that controlling my weight was really 80 percent what I ate and 20 percent how much I worked out. She added, "You will never be able to exercise away a bad diet."

"Food can be your anti-aging medicine."
— DEEPAK CHOPRA

And here's another gem from my father. He shared this nugget of wisdom with me when I was just a little girl, but I've always remembered it and hope you will too. My dad told me that as a physician, he often had patients turn to him for help with their weight. He said, "I always tell them that the best exercise is pushing yourself away from the table."

■ ■ ■ ■

PART THREE: SOUL

■ ■ ■ ■

"The soul always knows what to do to heal itself. The challenge is to silence the mind."
— CAROLINE MYSS

CHAPTER 17
WILL IT MATTER
FIVE YEARS FROM NOW?

"That the birds fly overhead, this you
cannot stop. That they build a nest in
your hair, this you can prevent."
— CHINESE PROVERB

If stress burned calories, I'd be a super-model. Okay, so maybe not, but if you took a poll of all the people standing in line at the supermarket checkout, how many of them do you think would say they feel stressed?

I think almost everyone!

A lot of people seem to be suffering from some type of stress these days. There are the big stressors, such as work, family, finances, health, and the state of our world. And then there are the smaller ones — the minutiae, not the least of which is what to make for dinner tonight and what to watch on Netflix.

It's easy to get caught up in life's little

dramas. But when we let ourselves get caught up in the *what ifs* of life, our focus can easily be drawn to what went wrong in a day or what could possibly go wrong tomorrow, and we forget to appreciate what actually went right. Sometimes we need to be reminded that having a bad moment, a bad day, or even a bad week doesn't mean we have a bad life.

> "I've been through some terrible things in my life, some of which actually happened."
> — MARK TWAIN

We aren't always aware of our stress, it's not like we can see it, but we sure can feel it. Sometimes it's a hidden fear driving our anxiety or anticipation of something that hasn't happened yet. It can wear us down, not just physically and mentally, but spiritually too. It can leave us with a short fuse in times when we need patience and thoughtfulness.

Sure, you won that battle with your sister-in-law and it felt great to tell your co-worker what you think of him, but where does that get us in the end? I would suggest that in most cases it only adds to our stress. I know when I've gotten into loggerheads with one of my kids, I can feel totally wiped out afterward. (Note to self: Don't engage! Or as my husband always says, "I don't negotiate with terrorists.") Although I don't remember teaching our kids, they are quite good at it. But, then again, just because I can't remember it doesn't mean I didn't do it.

I believe that just because stress is inevitable in life, it doesn't mean that we have to be a victim of it. We can learn to identify and deal with our stressors so that we can begin to make wiser decisions about how to stop them from wreaking all kinds of havoc. I've begun to identify when I'm feeling stressed earlier in the process and have found that by acknowledging its onset, I can then *decide* not to react to it when it hits and not allow myself to get all twisted into a knot. It's been an amazing discovery.

So what's been stressing you out? Is it your job? Is it your relationships? Is it your kids? Is it managing an aging parent? Or your finances? Is it making decisions? Is it being alone? How about the fear of losing your independence? To deal with our stresses, we must be able to identify them.

This isn't always so easy for everyone, so seems only fair that I should go first. Here's a glimpse into the kinds of things that sometimes worry and stress me out:

- Will my cancer come back?
- Do I look older? More like my mom?
- Am I making the right decisions with my teenage kids? Do I have the stamina to tell them no and stick to it? I don't want to screw them up!
- Am I handling my finances wisely? Have I planned for my future?
- Is my latest haircut as bad as I think it is? How long will it take to grow out?
- Will I finish this book on time and will it be well received?

Phew. I think I feel better now. Okay, I'm lying. I have at least fifty more I haven't shared.

Not only is it important to know what is stressing us out; we must also understand what stress can do to us on a deeper level. The stress response in humans is something called *fight-or-flight*. It's that physical response to anything that threatens us. We've all been there — we've *all* felt stress.

The heart begins to pump faster, our blood pressure rises, our breathing quickens, and our muscles tighten, and that's just the beginning. Odd how close these physical manifestations are to sexual arousal, but

290

that's the subject for another book, *Why Did I Get into This Bed?*

Stress may seem like an invisible health hazard, but it is harming us in ways that are increasingly hard to ignore. It certainly shows up in our nation's health care costs. Some experts estimate it's become a $1 *trillion* health epidemic. That's more expensive than the costs of treating cancer, smoking, diabetes, and heart disease combined. Look at some of these statistics from the CDC. They are not only mind-blowing, they're downright scary.

- Stress is a factor in five out of the six leading causes of death — heart disease, cancer, stroke, lower respiratory disease, and accidents.
- 43 percent of all adults suffer adverse health effects from stress.
- 75 to 90 percent of all doctor's office visits are for stress-related ailments and complaints.
- Chronic stress is now believed to be linked to depression in those who are susceptible to it.

So if you find that you're constantly sick and can't shake it, or that you are worn down emotionally as well as physically, it may be time to take a long, hard look at the stress in your life and how you might eliminate some of it. We're not going to be able to avoid all stress, but chronic stress can spell real trouble, especially if it continues into our later years. Here are some steps that we can all take to short-circuit many daily stresses.

Plan Your Work and Work Your Plan

I'm notorious for my to-do lists. My husband might make fun of them (admittedly, I can be a *little* neurotic about my lists), but they keep me focused and organized as opposed to being frazzled and harried. I keep a giant calendar in the kitchen. Everything that anyone in our home is scheduled to do is on that *mother of all calendars.* For me, being mentally prepared eliminates many potentially stressful moments in my life. Even if your kids are grown and out of the house, a calendar like this can keep you focused on your priority tasks for the day, week, or month ahead.

I'm also big on the concept of making mornings easier, deciding the night before what I have scheduled for the next day and what I should wear. This nightly ritual is a huge morning stress reliever. If I'm travelling, I pack ahead of time for upcoming trips. Basically, I try to *get ahead* of all the possible stressful moments in my life.

Have more than a busy day coming up? A chaotic workweek perhaps? Plan for that in advance too. It helps to reduce stress to spend a little quiet time on Sunday getting yourself prepared. Gym bag packed? Check. Work laptop and phone charged? Check. Important presentation proofed and ready to go? Check. Business lunch reservations made? Theater tickets purchased for Thursday date night with hubby or your bestie? Check, check. Try it for yourself. This method has proven to be a lifesaver for me.

Weekends can also be stressful because they are often filled with social obligations and parties that require gifts and cards. My method for avoiding a last-minute party panic is buying multiple gifts at one time. I usually watch for sales and buy several of the same items, so I always have something special on hand to bring with me. When my kids were little, this meant buying toys for all ages, but I find the method works for birthdays or anniversaries for girlfriends and relatives. When I find a clever gift that I would enjoy receiving myself, I buy a couple, have them wrapped, and the next time I'm running out to a birthday lunch, I'm not stressed out because of being caught empty-handed! Just make sure to put a sticky note on it to label what it is . . . otherwise, all that wrapping will be a waste! Trust me on this one. How embarrassing would it be for a friend to get an iTunes gift card and some glitter shadow while your granddaughter gets a new pair of reading glasses complete with a necklace to hold them.

The same holds true for finding the perfect greeting card. Who among us hasn't been late to a party because we've had to stop on the way for a card? Ugh! I solved that problem a long time ago by creating a card file for every possible occasion. Whenever I find myself in a store where cards are sold and I have a few extra minutes to spare, I stock up. I actually find the card aisle an oddly calming place. Without fail, a few of the cards will always make me chuckle. Need a card? Just come to my house.

Here are a few other ideas I think will go a long way toward cutting down on the age-accelerating stress we all seem to encounter in our fast-paced lives.

Unplug

Do you find that these days when you meet up with friends for lunch or coffee, they are frequently checking their phones or scrolling through their social media?! It drives me crazy. I think we should put a special value on real face-to-face communications, don't you? And don't get me started on teens and their technology. Every time I see their heads tilted downward, eyes locked on their phones, and their thumbs fast at work, it worries me to no end. I keep telling them that there is actually a physical toll to be paid for plugging into technology 24/7. The fact is that the human head weighs about 12 pounds and every inch your head tilts forward can make it feel another 10 pounds heavier. The result can be sagging shoulders, sore necks, bad posture and possibly even degenerative disc disease. And that's the physical impact.

I also worry about the emotional impact it can have on them. The truth is, this is a mounting concern for a lot of us. By the way, I know plenty of adults who are equally addicted to their devices.

> "My wife tried to look up ADD on WebMD but ended up on Pinterest.
> Now she's making a wreath while fixing dinner and origami-folding the laundry."
> — UNKNOWN

A lot of research has been done on the

benefits of unplugging to destress. Many spas are now offering sessions on digital detoxing. It's been shown that when people unplug at home after work, they feel fresher and recharged the next morning. People who unplug say they spend more time with family and friends, have better communication in interpersonal relationships, and exercise more frequently. One way to cut down on the distraction of technology is to turn off notifications. That constant pinging and vibrating can take you away from the moment in the real world you could be enjoying. And all too often it can send you down that tech rabbit hole we all know too well. Haven't you ever clicked on something you think will take only a second to read, and thirty minutes later — okay, maybe an hour — you're still engrossed. You've forever lost that time and the live interactions you could have had in the interim, because you got sucked into some Internet site.

"I'd like to introduce you to Pinterest. But first take a moment to say goodbye to all your family and friends."
— UNKNOWN

With apps and social media came an entirely different kind of stressor than we've ever experienced before: FOMO or Fear of Missing Out. Young people are especially vulnerable, but they are, by no means, alone in this phenomenon. Constantly seeing what fabulous things your friends are doing has been found to produce a recurring state of anxiety for many.

Hey, maybe this is where aging is an advantage, since we tend to be more willing to stay home, relax, and be with our loved ones.

For those who sleep with their phones right next to them (by the way, surveys indicate 44 percent of us do just that!), the blue light from the screens can make it difficult for our body to fall asleep. So for a good, sound, uninterrupted night's slumber, try plugging in your phone somewhere where the screen is not visible to you or you can unplug altogether. Your dreams will be more pleasant and your sleep far more restful!

Putting our phones down more often during waking hours will also give our eyes a break from eye strain, our neck a chance to relax, our hands a break from scrolling and texting, and our mind a chance to be in the moment in the real world.

"I saw a guy at Starbucks today.
No iPhone. No tablet. No laptop.
He just sat there.
Drinking coffee.
Like a psychopath."

— UNKNOWN

Take a Bath

I once read that life is like a hot bath. It feels good while we're in it, but the longer we stay, the more wrinkles we get. But really, who doesn't love a hot bath? I find that whenever I light a few candles, put some scented bath salts in my tub (or Epsom salts if my muscles are feeling achy), and I stretch out, it's hard to make myself get out of the tub before I end up looking like a prune!

There is much science behind this hot bath suggestion. Heat gets our blood moving, which is good for our circulation and can help ease sore or tight muscles. Adding Epsom salts can reduce inflammation in our joints too. Taking a warm bath also helps reduce our blood pressure, which can help prevent more serious heart conditions, including a heart attack or stroke. Soaking in warm water causes our body temperature to increase and our blood vessels to dilate, so it's said to be helpful in removing toxins and relieving anxiety. I love it because it also acts as a natural decongestant, which could help relieve sinus problems and colds. Most of all, I feel as if I am surrendering all of my worries in the tub. So taking that warm bath isn't just a luxury, it can hold many bodily and emotional health benefits.

And finally, I just have to tell you about one other theory. It is suggested that being submerged in warm liquid is comforting because it gives us the feeling of being in the womb, which induces a sense of security that can permit our mind and our body to relax. Personally, I can't relate to that one, because the thought of being squished inside a womb sounds totally claustrophobic. But that's just me.

Exercise

It almost seems a little cruel to follow a hot bath suggestion by recommending exercise, so I apologize. However, exercise can go a long way in providing peace of mind. When people suffer from stress and anxiety, they often think they need medicine to help them cope but exercising is actually considered as powerful as some drugs.

Cortisol is a stress hormone that is released in our body when we are feeling anxious. Movement depletes cortisol and therefore combats anxiety. Would you believe that just 10 minutes of physical activity can help stave off or relieve stress? It's true. A simple walk around your neighborhood could do the trick. Or even a walk around the nearest mall — sorry, my mind just naturally goes there.

> "Cinderella is proof that a new pair of shoes can change your life."
>
> — UNKNOWN

You might question whether a 10-minute stroll can really have a positive impact, but according to the ADAA (Anxiety and Depression Association of America) psychologists studying how exercise relieves anxiety and depression suggest that a 10-minute walk may actually be as good as a 45-minute workout. That news alone should relieve some of your tensions!

Exercise not only helps reduce stress and anxiety, it can help us maintain a healthy hormone balance and a strong immune system. There is significant evidence that increased levels of anxiety can weaken our immune system, our body's defense mechanism against disease-causing microorganisms. A weakened immune system can leave us vulnerable if we come into contact with bacteria or viruses.

So finding a form of exercise that we like is important. There are several activities that are actually considered *happiness-inducing* exercises. (Of course, you should only engage in exercises that are appropriate for your physical condition.)

Hiking: Going for a hike in the outdoors can lower our stress levels, much more than taking a walk in the city can, because spending time in nature itself is a mood-booster.

Yoga: By its very nature, yoga emphasizes deep breathing and internal focus, which can help us to destress *and* find peace of mind. Yoga helps us reason with our thoughts and let go of them accordingly.

Weight Training: People usually associate strength training with building muscle; however, strength training can also reduce stress, improve our mood, and help regulate our sleep. Lifting weights not only lifts our spirits, it can give us chiseled arms that look great in T-shirts, and that, my friends, should be a real mood enhancer.

Fun Dance Class: This one is my favorite! Whether you choose a Zumba class or you

301

just put on some music and get your groove on in the privacy of your own home, dancing is a terrific way to relieve stress and anxiety.

The higher the intensity of your dance workout, the more benefit you can receive and the more you can elevate your spirits. So when you start to feel your stomach in a knot, put on some music and take a quick whirl around your living room. Getting your Ginger Rogers on may be just the right remedy.

Eat Breakfast: Okay, I know this one sounds so basic, and I don't think I ever associated eating breakfast with reducing stress, but apparently a morning meal kickstarts our metabolism for the day and also helps stabilize our blood sugar level, which is what helps lower stress and helps keep us balanced.

If we skip eating a good breakfast, our body may not be able to handle the kinds of conditions and events that bring on stress. Whenever we are in stressful situations, our body produces certain hormones. These hormones make the body lose some essential nutrients, such as calcium, zinc, iron, and magnesium. A good breakfast can supply all of these essential nutrients, allowing us to better cope with stress. Breakfast can also help maintain the level of antioxidants in our body, which play a major role in avoiding the side effects of stress, such as mood swings.

A breakfast that contains some carbohydrates can also help us maintain a good mood. These foods all help in sending the amino acid tryptophan into the brain. Tryptophan increases the production of serotonin, which is a mood lifter and a stress-busting hormone.

We can also add an orange or a banana to our breakfast, as oranges contain vitamin C, which is also a mood enhancer, and a banana can help keep us feeling full throughout the day.

After fasting all night long, we really don't want to skip breakfast. As you can see, our body needs this meal, rich in vitamin C, antioxidants, minerals, and carbohydrates, which all play important roles in supercharging our metabolism, increasing our energy level, and enhancing our ability to focus, think clearly, and stay calm. Without it, we're all prone to getting *hangry*! Confession: I learned that word from my kids.

Limit Caffeine and Soda: Caffeine has been found to have a number of health benefits; however, it can also affect our body in ways that increase our anxiety, interfere with our sleep, and prevent us from optimally managing stress. Many people depend on their morning java to fuel them for the day. Coffee is well-known for its ability to increase our alertness, but when consumed in larger amounts, it can lead to a nervous edginess. Too much coffee can have an effect on our body that is similar to stress and can also impact our hormones, causing our adrenal glands to stop producing adrenaline. Adrenaline is that fight-or-flight hormone we spoke about earlier, which triggers our immediate stress response.

One of caffeine's most sought-after qualities is its ability to help us stay awake. Just ask any college student. But conversely, too much caffeine can interfere with our sleep. Studies have found that high caffeine intake appears to increase the amount of time it takes to fall asleep and can also decrease total sleep time, especially in the elderly.

Of course, we may not even realize that too much caffeine is interfering with our sleep, if we aren't keeping track of just how much we're taking in. Coffee and tea are the most concentrated sources of caffeine; however, it's also found in soda, cocoa, energy drinks, and a few types of medication. The amount of caffeine we can consume without affecting our sleep is individual; it depends on our genetics and other factors. It's also important that we be aware of how much caffeine we are consuming late in the day because its effects can take several hours to wear off. Research shows that caffeine remains in our system for an average of five hours; however, that time period could range from one to nine hours, depending on the individual.

It's up to us to monitor how much caffeine our body can tolerate, but if we're feeling edgy or having trouble sleeping, it's likely that we should be cutting back coffee and soda consumption.

Just Breathe: When you start to feel yourself getting uptight, try to stop, stretch, and take a few breaths. Breathing exercises are a great way to relax, reduce tension, and relieve stress. I've done a number of breathing sessions with Beth Bielat, a fitness trainer who is also a Lifebreath trainer. I've learned some easy breathing techniques from Beth that can truly stop stress and anxiety in their path.

Deep breathing: This kind of breathing activates the parasympathetic nervous system, which is sometimes referred to as the *brakes* for stress. Essentially, breathing deeply sends a message to our brain to chill out, and then the brain broadcasts that message to the rest of our body.

Deep breathing can be used anywhere or anytime, and no one will be the wiser. Visualizing something calming at the same time can also help. Some people like to think of a sun-kissed, white sand beach or a bright green meadow as they inhale and exhale slowly. I love to use colors to guide me. I imagine blue, sparkling, fresh, clean, quiet air, which I associate with joy and good health, as I breathe in, and bright red or purple air, which I associate with stress and sadness, as I breathe out. You might even visualize your stressful thoughts being expelled or booted from your body, observing it without judgement. Can you already see how this works? Tell me the truth: Did you just exhale robustly while thinking of . . . you fill in the blank; I don't want to get into trouble!

Diaphragmatic or Belly Breathing:
Stress is usually accompanied by shallow breathing in the upper chest. We can reduce stress by consciously breathing using our diaphragm. Belly breathing helps relieve

tension and increases blood flow. When every deep breath goes straight to our lungs, filling our body with oxygen, it helps to control the nervous system and encourage our body to relax more. The net effect is that we feel way more confident. Here are a few easy steps to learn this breathing technique.

1. Lie on your back on your bed, on the floor, or perhaps on a lounge chair in your yard where the air is fresh and bright. Place a pillow under your head and one under your knees.
2. Place one hand on your belly. Now breathe in through your nose, and as you breathe in, feel your belly rise as it fills with air. (Think of what a newborn baby's belly looks like when it breathes.)
3. Now exhale through your nose. Repeat this several times.

Pursed-Lip Breathing: This was the first breathing technique I learned while on my ascent up the Grand Tetons. I was struggling with my breathing as we tackled a steep incline at about 10,000 feet. One of the climbing guides noticed that I was short of breath and said I'd have an easier time with the climb if I used pursed-lip breathing. He taught me how to do it right there on the mountainside, and as soon as I caught on, it helped. This technique works just as well when you're climbing stairs or carrying heavy bags from the grocery store and feel stressed and short of breath. Here are a few easy steps to learn the pursed lip breathing technique.

1. Plant your feet firmly on the floor.
2. Shake out, then relax the muscles in your neck and shoulders.
3. Inhale through your nose or mouth for 2 counts.
4. As you breathe in, feel your belly expanding.
5. Purse your lips as if you're about to whistle, blow out a candle, or kiss me for teaching you these relaxing exercises. Then exhale.
6. Breathe out until all the air is gone and your belly is no longer extended. A good way to be sure that you are fully exhaling is to take twice as long to breathe out as you've taken to breathe in.

Calming Breathing: Here is a basic

breathing technique that is, in essence, like a new version of *counting to 10* when you're stressed out.

1. Take a long, slow breath in through your nose, remaining aware of how your lower portion of your lungs are filling, followed by your upper lungs.
2. Hold that deep breath to a count of three.
3. Breath out slowly through pursed lips while you relax your facial muscles, jaw, shoulders, chest, and stomach.

Square Breathing: This is a simple breathing technique that some people find helpful because it has a visual component to it that helps you focus better. There is also a rhythm to it as it's based on a four-count breathing cycle. Here's how it works.

1. Visualize a square frame in your mind. Focus on the lower left corner.
2. Inhale for four counts while moving your gaze to the upper left corner.
3. Hold your breath for another four counts while you bring your gaze

309

across the top to the upper right corner.

4. Exhale for four counts as you move your gaze down to the lower right corner.
5. Now hold your breath for another four counts as you bring your gaze back across to the lower left corner where you started.
6. Repeat as necessary.

One question a lot of people have is whether it's better to breathe through your mouth or your nose. I was trained to breathe in through my nose and out through my mouth. But when I researched this, I learned that exhaling through the nose, which is smaller than the mouth, creates greater air pressure and slower exhalation, which gives the lungs extra time to extract a greater amount of oxygen.

These are all doable, right? They are great tools to have in your anti-stress, age-proofing toolbox. And here's the best news: In addition to these breathing techniques, we also have a set of inner resources that we can all call upon to manage and alleviate our stress. They include courage, optimism, humility, humor, joy, acceptance, forgiveness, love, and, oh yes, patience. These inner resources are to our souls what medicine is to our bodies. I like to think of these as my *inner muscles.*

And imagine this: The more we strengthen these inner muscles, the more we can count on them in our next challenging moment, which will no doubt be sometime later today.

> "Most of the shadows of this life are caused by our standing in our own sunshine."
> — UNKNOWN

Sometimes averting stress is just a matter of realigning our expectations in life. Should we really be expecting our busy boss to stop and give thanks to us for work well done? Perhaps they've noticed our fine performance but are in the middle of juggling a million other stress-inducing responsibilities of their own. Should we really be expecting our mate to automatically know what pressures we faced during our day? Well . . .

While you have heard this truism from me before in slightly different terms, there is a nuance to it that is worth exploring further: Stress is not really something that happens to us. Rather it is how we *react* to what happens. Whoa! Wait a minute! Did we just discover that *we* bring on our own stress by how we respond to certain situations and therefore we can manage our stress by controlling or changing our responses? Let's take a moment to be empowered by that statement. It's almost as if we're one step ahead of everyone around us who haven't yet learned this crucial life secret.

Understanding that we create or perpetuate so much of our own stress, and that all too often the circumstances don't warrant our strong reaction, is actually enlightening and heartening. Isn't it? I think it is. With this knowledge, we can short circuit our stress reaction and save ourselves a lot of angst and headaches.

Stress does not go with my outfit.
— UNKNOWN

So the next time you feel like strangling the living $#@ out of someone, remember that you're the one who actually suffers from your anger. It's sort of like drinking poison and hoping the other person dies. Developing this kind of emotional maturity allows us to accept our feelings, and then let them go so that we can move on and focus on the next moment of our lives . . . very likely a better moment.

"Dear Stress, I think it's time we break up. Love, Me"

— UNKNOWN

CHAPTER 18
LIFE WOULD BE EASIER WITH PIÑATAS PLACED THROUGHOUT THE DAY

"Learning to ignore things is one of the great paths to inner peace."
— ROBERT J. SAWYER,
AUTHOR OF *CALCULATING GOD*

Have you ever had a day like this? Your alarm clock didn't go off; you burned your bagel; you couldn't find your car keys; morning traffic was excruciatingly slow; work was crazy busy — and now you're back in the evening rush hour. When the stresses start to pile on like this, that's when the theory of *not reacting* gets tested.

I remember when I first learned about the concept of *non-reactive behavior* in a book called *Wherever You Go, There You Are,* by Jon Kabat-Zinn. I felt I had discovered something so profound it would change my life. It is the idea that reacting to a person or a situation is not a bodily function, but rather a choice of ours.

314

I find this idea is so fundamental to living a better quality of life at any age that I've actually read Kabat-Zinn's book twice, maybe even three times. Its title refers to the notion that even though we all travel through the same world, each of us is affected by it differently because we are seeing it through our own particular lens.

It's as if we are wearing a customized pair of glasses that have lenses containing everything that has ever happened to us and every belief that we've ever drawn from our life's experiences. The result is that wherever we go in life, we view the scene before us through our own personal prism, with all its preconceptions, biases, disappointments, and hopes.

"Life is the movie you see through your
own unique eyes.
Your emotions color what you see.
It makes little difference what's happening
out there.
It's how you take it all in that counts."
— DENIS WAITLEY

Another one of my favorite mindfulness authors and teachers is Brian Luke Seaward. When I started exploring inner peace and mindfulness, Brian's book *Stand Like Moun-*

tain, Flow like Water changed how I looked at human behavior and our responsibility in it.

Brian (I'm allowed to call him by his first name since we've become friends) teaches us that if we take a step back rather than charge right in and get emotionally involved whenever we are confronted with stressful situations — even when they're piled on — we have an opportunity to think about what we'd like the end result to be. This approach allows us to take a breather and can help us avoid stress and its many consequences when we do react. Perhaps, if at one point in that crazy day I just described, we just took a breather, collected our wits, and thought before we acted at each turn, we could have avoided some of the other things that when awry. What if it was as simple as thinking that it was *not* a doomed day after one or two mishaps?

What an easier, calmer world this would be if we all approached life's annoying moments this way — if we all just took a beat and refrained from spontaneously reacting.

"We are the only creatures on earth who can change our biology by what we think and feel."
— DEEPAK CHOPRA

In another of Brian Luke Seaward's books, *Stressed Is Desserts Spelled Backward,* he shows us how, in the same way eating a sugary dessert can spiral into an emotional high, letting ourselves get sucked into a stress-filled moment can spiral into an emotional low, inducing more sadness, anger, and frustration. Having an understanding of how our body works and learning how not to react can really help stop that downward spiral in its tracks, enabling us to fend off stress and increase joy in our life.

Once I realized that stress was not something that happened to me, but rather something I could control by how I responded to negative situations, my life was transformed. What an *aha* moment. I began experimenting with this concept, and sure enough, I found that I really did have the power to pause and make the choice not to *go there* — to actually stop the stress before it ever overtook my day or my life. That was perhaps one of the most important discoveries I've ever made. Spoiler alert: While the art of non-reactive behavior is life-changing, it's also much harder than it sounds. But it is definitely worth learning.

"When we are no longer able to change a

situation, we are challenged to change ourselves."

— VICTOR FRANKL

Okay, if the idea of stepping back and reflecting doesn't float your boat, maybe it would be easier to imagine piñatas strategically placed throughout your day ready for a good whack when you feel stressed. One whack . . . that's all it would take to diffuse the stressful energy these incidents stir. Oh, I'm calmer already. I can move on now. Can't you just feel the relief? Wouldn't that solve a lot and save so much emotional stress? I thought I'd list a few moments when having a piñata to pop might come in handy, along with some ideas about how to avoid the stress in the absence of an actual candy-stuffed papier-mâché donkey and a stick.

Piñata Moment #1: Consumed by Worry
Ready for a life-changing revelation? Get this: Worrying won't stop bad stuff from happening. Imagine that. All worrying does is stop us from enjoying the good stuff.

For this reason, we need to *stop worrying now!* Without even knowing it, we are often coloring everything we see, putting our spin on it, creating problems for ourselves that might not otherwise exist. I'll admit it; I've worried that certain people didn't like me, when later I learned they were just intimidated and simply shied away. I've stressed when my husband didn't call back after we'd had words, only to discover that he was in the middle of dealing with a big business issue. He wasn't even thinking about our last call. (That's a guy for you.) He'd already let the issue go, and there I was still stewing over it, feeling hurt. (That's an emotional female for you.) Makes me think I want to be a guy in my next life, so I could just sail through rough waters focused on what I needed to do and not so much on the perceptions of others. Maybe I wouldn't even need piñatas.

Piñata Moment #2: Contending with Conflicting Priorities

Know your *priorities* and stick to them. This might be the most important life strategy that I can recommend in order to eliminate a lot of life's stress and live more joyfully. But with that, I will also note that it can be a difficult rule to follow. First of all, we need to be honest with ourselves. What are our priorities? It might sound like a simple question, but when was the last time you asked yourself this?

319

For all of my adult life, I struggled to navigate the conflicting priorities of a working mom. When my three older girls were little and I was working on morning TV, I was always questioning whether I had the right priorities and the right balance. One day a friend told me that Howard Stern, the radio shock jock, had been ripping me apart on his show saying something like, "What's up with this Joan Lunden supposedly being some kind of a Super Mom? We all know she's not with her kids in the morning, waking them up, getting them ready for school. She's not smiling at them and kissing them goodbye; she's smiling at us and telling us the news." When I heard that, as you can imagine, it made me second-guess the entire way I had structured my life. Was I doing it all wrong? A flood of stress washed over me.

I was fully aware that my unusual early morning work hours made me miss the wake-up routine; however, those hours also got me back at home much earlier than most people. I always felt like that was the trade-off for putting my feet on the carpet at 3:30 every morning. But I will admit Howard Stern really got to me, and after that, I couldn't help but feel a little guilty about not being home in the mornings.

Without even realizing it, I had let Howard's expectations of what a mother's priorities should be affect my opinion of myself as a parent. Clearly, I couldn't be there in the early mornings, since I worked at a morning show. Yet you know what? My girls never knew anything different. Their mommy was on the TV screen in the kitchen when they were at the breakfast table. And by the way, they always watched, even if it was just to see what Mommy was wearing that day. And oh yes, they kissed Mommy goodbye on the TV. Being there for wake up simply wasn't possible, but we all made the best of it and crafted our own morning ritual to fondly reflect back on.

I get that Howard's job is to poke fun and provoke a response. And we all know how darn good he is at it. While I was working on GMA, I belonged to a small gym that was directly across the street from our studio. I'd go there to work out after the show. Occasionally, I'd see this super tall guy working out, too, and I couldn't get over how much he looked like Howard Stern. One day I asked my trainer who the guy was. "That's Howard Stern," my trainer said, as if to imply, "Who else would it be?" I wondered in that moment, *Do I say something to him about his characterization of me as a mom?* Nah. I'd let it go. Besides, he was a parent, too, who also worked mornings. I think he had first-hand knowledge of the situation. In the end, I don't believe our work made either of us bad parents. If anything, it allowed us to be better parents because we cherished the times we did spend with our children even more. At least I know that's how I feel. Even Howard has come around, recently talking about how he treated people unkindly over the years and now regrets it. It's never too late to change.

For the record, after I left the morning show and was finally at home for that whole wake-up and get the-kids-ready-for-school routine, I must tell you . . . I think it's highly overrated.

We all have to decide what our priorities are, not only what's important to us but what's realistic. Think about it. Have you taken on more than you can possibly do? Are you trying to continue working in addition to taking care of your grandchildren or your elderly parents? Is taking care of a home and getting dinner on the table at night also on that list? Lots of people are finding themselves in that position, and all too often, they end up sick because they're not caring for themselves.

Studies show that women tend to manage it all by reducing sleep and eliminating personal time. But remember, those strategies take a toll on our health.

Piñata Moment #3:
Feeling as If There Aren't Enough Hours
in the Day!
Running life by the seat of our pants is a sure-fire way for us to burn. I've always found that I get the most frazzled, bitchy, and schizo (to use some clinical terms) when I haven't properly planned and kept my life in order. *A little organization in life will go a long way.* When my life feels like it is in order, I feel like I can get more done. And when I get more done, I feel more fulfilled and more in control.

My Filofax used to assure my sanity — remember those? They were replaced by smartphones. Despite my complaints about the kids being too attached to their phones, nowadays I can't function without mine. Like most people, my life is contained in that damn device. Admittedly, I love that I have every address, birthday, and task at my fingertips.

But keeping order in our lives requires more than keeping a good calendar. An even more important step is determining which tasks in life are really necessary, and which ones are optional. Honestly, how often does that junk drawer in our kitchen *really* need to be organized? I remember Erma Bombeck, a wonderful humorist who was a guest on GMA for years, saying, "Cleaning our house while our kids are still growing is like shoveling the walk before it stops snowing."

It's really a matter of paying attention to what most pushes our buttons. For me it's usually the last-minute scramble, but for you it may be something different. The object is not to suffer through that stressful moment only to go through it again next time. We need to identify what it is and take a moment to figure out how to minimize it.

Candidly, for many years I kept repeating the same stressful scenarios without stopping to fix them. I hit a point where I knew I had to find a way to rid myself of those recurring frustrations. It took some doing, but I learned to delegate a little. (I'm not a *complete* control freak . . . only a little bit of one . . . just ask my husband! On second thought, maybe not.)

One of those frustrating situations always began with the question, "What's for dinner?" It's such an innocent question, but one that can send a person into panic mode if you are the one responsible for getting dinner on the table after a full day of work.

Cooking several meals at one time on a quiet Sunday afternoon means extra meals ready to pop in the oven on a busy weeknight. Weekly menu planning can also help minimize the nightly decision-making and last-minute prepping. Buying pre-cut veggies also saves time on weeknights and may make it more likely to eat them. Some of you with the same challenges might also enjoy trying a meal delivery service on occasion. The service essentially shops and preps; you just cook! There are so many delicious ones to choose from now. The point is, we need to identify our stress triggers.

What stressors send you off the rails? And what steps could you take to alleviate them?

Piñata Moment #4: Wrestling with Multitasking Mania

Do you pride yourself on being a multi-tasker? Me too. But all too often it leaves me feeling like my brain has too many tabs open. Confession: Sometimes it's almost like a personal challenge — just how many things can I do at once? For the record, I can brush my teeth, pee, and change the toilet roll all at the same time! Aren't you proud of me? It can leave me feeling pretty full of myself.

What's worse is that the only time I ever hurt myself, or drop and break things, is when I'm trying to do two things at once or carry five things upstairs.

Are you afflicted with this same multitasking obsession? Do you really think you can read and watch TV at the same time? How about texting while in a meeting or out to dinner with your spouse? (Maybe you should ask your spouse what they think about that.)

Many people would say that we get more done by multitasking, right? The truth is, the brain is wired to do only one thing at a time. We might *think* that we're multitasking, but science will tell us that we're really not doing two things at once, but rather two individual things in rapid succession.

Psychologists who study the mental process say that we are mono-taskers. When we take on several tasks at once, it doesn't expand the brain's capacity to accomplish both; it simply increases the brains cognitive load (the amount of mental effort it must put out) and the result is that we simply reduce the attention we give to each of the tasks.

It seems the smartest approach to tackling the tasks in a day is not to do more, but to do what matters the most at any given time.

Multitasking has a tendency to make all tasks seem equally important as we are taking them on, which lessens our ability to consider each task more carefully. This issue of wading through our daily tasks has become more and more challenging as we've added the constant interaction with our electronic devices.

Piñata Moment #5: Inundated by Inbox Insanity

It is estimated that over 200 billion email messages are sent each day worldwide. I read that if all of those emails were printed and stacked, the pile would be 12,000 miles high! Can you imagine? Because the Internet allows anyone to reach us at any given time, we are bombarded with headlines, both good and bad, from sunrise to sunset. Most of us are not even aware of how much this is impacting us.

Medical experts warn that our constant interaction with the Internet can end up creating a sense of isolation for some people, which can negatively impact their health and certainly their happiness. This next generation often seems to be more focused on touching their screens and their keyboards than touching other people! How will this affect their ability to form meaningful relationships? I think that worries all of us, doesn't it?

So how about you? How many emails are in your inbox? I just looked at my inbox and I have over 200, and what's worse is that I just spent a plane ride from California to New York cleaning it out! I just can't seem to ever get ahead of it. So I looked for ways to cut back on my digital clutter and found some great tips that have really helped me.

1. Cut back on those notifications from Facebook, Twitter, and any other social media platforms that constantly compete for our attention. Basically, anything that goes *ping* in the night.
2. Limit how many people you allow yourself to follow on your social media platforms.
3. Don't buy or download apps you don't really need. I have to confess to this one, and what's worse, I was paying a monthly fee for apps that I wasn't using. I'm proud to say that I just deleted them all!
4. Three words: *Un. Sub. Scribe.* I mean it; periodically schedule time to clean out your inbox and unsub-

scribe from extraneous newsletters.

5. Organize your emails in folders so you don't leave hundreds of read emails in your inbox.

6. Let things go. If you have been saving a newsletter, marking it as *unread* or *starred* but haven't bothered to read it yet, *delete it*! If it's that important and you think of it later, you'll google it!

7. Don't let incoming emails sidetrack you. If you're in deep on a project and an email pops up, don't feel compelled to open it and lose focus on the task you're concentrating on. Sandra Chapman, founder and chief director of the Center for BrainHealth, recommends scheduling "work time" where you only concentrate on a task or project at hand and intermittent breaks to catch up on emails, phone calls, and so on. This will allow you to more fully focus on what you need to get done.

Piñata Moment #6: Overwhelmed by Clutter

I'm a little old school so I tend to write things down, which means my desk can

329

often be cluttered with scraps of paper . . . lots of scraps. I don't like disarray, so I often find myself pushing all the sticky notes and the junk mail I don't know what to do with into my desk drawer. Every time I open that drawer, I am appalled at how messy I've let it become. Yet I continually take out what I need — and then I close it! I'll get to it someday, right? Yeah, right.

Well, one day I decided that it was ridiculous to let the chaos of that drawer cause me one more day of stress. Just do it, Joan! I decided the best way for me to tackle that drawer and any other little projects around my house was to treat them like business appointments and schedule them on my calendar.

Now I had a date with my desk drawer. Admittedly I also posted my commitment on Facebook so that I'd have some accountability! And it worked! I swear, cleaning out and organizing that desk drawer made me feel lighter and definitely less stressed.

It doesn't matter whether it is my inbox or my home files, when I know they are falling into disarray my nerves begin to fray. Sometimes we can't put our finger on what is bothering us, but messy homes and workspaces tend to leave most of us feeling anxious and overwhelmed. Yet rarely do we recognize clutter as a significant source of stress. Fortunately, though, clutter is one of the easiest life stressors to fix.

For me, one of the reasons why stuff piles up is because I simply have too much of it. Way too much! We hold onto things for a lot of different reasons. Sometimes we think we'll need it later. Sometimes we keep them just because we spent good money on them even if we haven't touched them in months or even years. For instance, I have lots and lots of books that I've bought over time that caught my eye in the bookstore but that I've never read. Books hold a certain reverence for me, and I keep them all, but now I don't have any more shelf space.

Turns out that there is real science behind our inability to let go of items that we attach ourselves to, even if we know that we will never use them. Researchers at Yale University identified two areas in our brain, the anterior cingulate cortex and insula, which are associated with pain, that also light up in response to letting go of items we own or feel some sort of connection to.

However, keeping excess stuff and letting it clutter our surroundings can have an impact on our ability to focus and process information. It overloads our senses, makes us feel stressed, and can even impair our ability to think creatively. Neuroscientists at Princeton University found that when they compared people's task performance — some in an organized environment, others in a disorganized environment — physical clutter competed for their attention, resulting in decreased performance and increased stress. The moral of that story: Declutter to de-stress.

Piñata Moment #7: Suffering from Separation Anxiety

One of my pet peeves is not being able to find a certain sweater when I want it. Why? Because my closet is filled with so many clothes I never wear that I can't always find my favorite things. Don't we all have way too many items like that? Why don't we just toss them? Truthfully, there's a part of me that just doesn't want to admit that I made a dumb impulse buy. Of course, these days I just blame impulse buys on my hormones.

It's always been a challenge for me to part with items, even if I know full well I'm not using them. Then I had an amazing awakening. I read Marie Kondo's *The Life-Changing Magic of Tidying Up*. At first, I thought the idea of touching everything in my home and asking it if it brought me joy was the kookiest thing I'd ever heard. Then I started doing it, and by God, stuff answered me back.

One day while cleaning out my underwear drawer, I swear one of my bras told me that my boobs looked a bit droopy when I wore it. You can bet I threw that bra right in the trash. The book then sent me on a scavenger hunt all over my house looking for other *red flags* — things I kept around for no good reason and points of disorganization that caused me to stress every time I looked at them. Suddenly, I felt compelled to de-clutter. I made my way through my home and then my office on a mission of search and toss, repeating to myself, *If you don't use it, lose it.*

When I looked at my belongings with this kind of a discerning eye, I started noticing piles of things I'd been unnecessarily keeping. Did I really think I was going to return to a recipe or an article I hadn't gotten around to reading yet? I must tell you, it felt so good to toss those magazines and the stack of sticky notes papering my desk. I'd obviously scribbled those notes in a hurry because I couldn't even read most of them. I'm really not a hoarder, but I did generate six huge black plastic garbage bags of trash just in my home office!

Do I have you thinking about all the items overflowing in your closets and drawers now too? Writing this chapter really motivated me. As soon as I finish writing this book, I intend to get busy chucking a lot more. Wait. Did I just let it slip that I'm procrastinating? Seriously, I find it overwhelming to think about getting rid of *all* the excess in my house. That part of my brain, what's it called again? Oh yeah, the anterior cingulate cortex, starts to twitch when I think about it. So even though Marie Kondo says to attack it all at once, I've decided to compartmentalize — you know, do that thing men are so good at doing — and take on one bookshelf or one drawer at a time. Or should I say, one piñata at a time?

Piñata Moment #8: Protecting Quality Family Time

In the days before cellphones and email, this piñata did not exist. Finding time for family and fun didn't used to be such a challenge. When we'd leave work in the evening, our time would be our own until we got to work the next morning. It was that black and white. Now I find that all 24 hours of my day are a *gray area.* When you get a business email in the middle of dinner, what is the protocol? Isn't that family time? It used to be.

I think it's become somewhat difficult in

today's fast-paced, electronically connected world to keep the different aspects of our lives balanced. We are constantly deluged with texts, emails, FB messages, tweets, LinkedIn articles, and exchanges — oh wait, I forgot Instagram and Pinterest too! This has all become a daily part of our lives, which is why we have to work hard to protect our non-work time.

It's so easy to get distracted, but our loved ones also need our attention. It's important for us to listen and to care about what went on during their day. Our families notice when we are tuned in to our electronics rather than being tuned in to them. We need to be present in the moment and frankly we need to unplug and recharge. It's important that we *protect quality time with our family . . . and also, time for* ourselves.

Piñata Moment #9: Craving Me Time

Taking time to care for ourselves can be a point of stress in most women's lives. Why is that? Why do we feel guilty or selfish when we do carve out that time? I've always felt that it's because we're wired differently than men and it's simply not in our nature to put ourselves first even for an hour or two. The truth is, if we take this much needed time for self-care we will be better mates, better moms, better friends, and better workers. This is one place where I think we could learn a little something from our fun-loving male counterparts who seem to be able to play a pick-up basketball game with guy friends after work, golf on the weekend, or sit and watch sports on TV whenever they want and not seem to feel guilty. If we could do that more easily, we wouldn't need this piñata.

Piñata Moment #10: Too Proud to Ask for Help

We could cut down on a lot of our daily stress if we just learned to ask for help. Come on, let's be honest though, we don't always let others lend a hand. Why do we limit ourselves this way? Obviously, it's because other people can't load the dishwasher or make a bed as well as we can. It's our nature to do it all ourselves, be martyrs, and be stressed out and exhausted, but I don't think most women realize what a toll that behavior is taking on our health and longevity.

And as shocking as it may seem, husbands and children are not mind readers, so they don't always know or intuit when we're feeling overwhelmed and want them to pitch in. We need to talk with our families about what it takes to operate as a team, how it's important for everyone to work together in that endeavor, and to find some kind of equitable sharing of tasks. If we just do it all ourselves and never have that discussion, then we'll always be overwhelmed and resentful, and they will always think we are one crabby lunatic.

Chapter 19
Mistakes and Regrets:
It's Time to Let Them Go!

"After all these years, I am still involved
in the process of self-discovery.
It's better to explore life and make
mistakes than to play it safe.
Mistakes are part of the dues one pays
for a full life."
— Sophia Loren

The phrase *letting go* may be overused to the point of being high in the running for "New Age cliché of the century." However, the practice of letting go is, without a doubt, one of the most powerful inward maneuvers. It is not about forgetting, but rather, about accepting.

Letting go means just what it says. It's an intention to stop holding on to anything, whether it be an idea, a regret, a thing, a person, an event, a view, or a desire.

Our minds are constantly evaluating our experiences, comparing them against other experiences, or often against expectations that we've created. We do this out of fear that we're not good enough, that bad things might happen, that good things won't last, that other people won't like us, or that we won't get our way. This mindset can produce a retort, which we later wish we could take back. It can leave us asking, *Why did I respond to that person like that, or why did I respond at all?*

"To respond immediately to an angry person is like throwing fuel on a fire."
— UNKNOWN

My mom used to remind my brother and me when we were growing up that it's usually the reply that causes the trouble. Isn't that so true? I actually experience this challenge in my own home. Teenagers can try a parent's patience, as you likely know, especially when they begin to assert themselves and find their own sense of independence. I've learned that if I reply to every eye roll or diss from one of my kids, I'm definitely just looking for trouble. It's not always easy, but I really make a concerted effort not to be hurt or let them push my buttons and respond.

The next time someone pushes your buttons, try not to listen to your ego — sit on your reply no matter how clever your comeback may be.

Whenever I think about the act of letting go, it always takes me back to an interview I did years ago when I was hosting *Good Morning America*. I spoke with thousands of people over my twenty years on that show, but I'll always remember one particular morning, sitting across from a woman named Virginia who was finally finding closure and peace after suffering an unimaginable tragedy. Her 12-year-old daughter had been brutally raped and killed, and the man who had committed the terrible crime was to be put to his death later that day.

As we began the interview, I noticed that she seemed calm and resolute, and I asked her how she was dealing with her grief and her anger and the man's impending execution. She told me how rage and anguish had completely consumed her life in the years following her daughter's murder. She also told me how her inability to cope with her sorrow and anger caused her marriage to fall apart. One day, as she wept to a friend, she asked over and over, "Why is this happening to me? Why can't I move on?" Her friend replied, "A heart filled with anger has no room for love."

Virginia said it was on that day that she let go of the rage and began to heal. She realized that while the murderer had taken her daughter's life, her own anger and sorrow were now taking her life. Her friend told her that she needed to stop focusing on her pain and begin to focus on the blessings in her life. Virginia couldn't change the events of the past, but by letting go of those negative emotions that had paralyzed and disempowered her, she would be free to begin living life again.

No matter how big or small our troubles are, if we can let them go, focus on possible solutions, and imagine a joyous future, we can take the first step toward finding peace within. Virginia had told me that she felt lighter as she headed home from speaking with her friend that day — as though a tremendous weight had been lifted from her heart. Instead of mourning the things that were missing in her life, she began to give thanks for her blessings, her health, her friends, and her new understanding that our thoughts create our reality. This is a message that she felt compelled to pass on to others who were dealing with grief.

And so, on that particular morning on GMA, Virginia was able to fondly remember her daughter's life, rather than dwell on her death. As for her daughter's killer, she said she was no longer holding on to any hatred towards him; she only felt pity.

That interview has stayed with me and so have the words that restored peace in Virginia's life, *A heart filled with anger has no room for love.* Virginia's profound ability to let go of her anger and sadness touched my life that morning. At the time of that interview, I was recently divorced and raising three young daughters. I knew all too well how easy it was to feel upset, overwhelmed, and alone. That morning, I, too, felt a weight lift from my heart, as I decided I would be far better off if I let go of the frustration and hurt feelings of the divorce so that I could find inner peace and embrace the possibilities of the future.

"How often do we allow a temporary defeat to affect us as if it were a permanent failure instead of learning from it and moving on?"
— NAPOLEON HILL

Letting go of heartaches, fears, regrets, and all the other layers of stress that we tend to carry around with us can have a profoundly positive impact on our lives and our happiness.

I've found that my healing has also taken the form of writing books. The more I give of myself through my writing and in helping others, the more peace and fulfillment I feel in my own life. Like Virginia, I also felt the need to pass on this life-altering message. By directing our minds, we direct our lives and ultimately create our own happiness.

"A day of worry is more exhausting than a week of work."
— UNKNOWN

I think our happiness in life greatly depends on our ability to navigate the bends in our road. I remember when in 1997, as I was leaving *Good Morning America* and contemplating what I was going to do next, my husband looked at me and said, "A bend in the road is not the end of the road, as long as you remember to make the turn."

Almost all of us have moments in our lives that seem to grab us by the neck and paralyze us with fear, anger, or hurt feelings. A fight with a friend or relative, receiving or spewing hurtful words that we wish we could take back, losing a job, or breaking up with a mate are all such moments. How we handle ourselves during these times can often affect the outcome.

I remember the day my agent called to tell me that ABC had decided to change the GMA hosts; they were going to hire younger ones.

I was being replaced.

That is a phrase that can knock the wind right out of you. It took a moment to even process the reality of it. Then came a flood of emotions. The first was humiliation. It was such a public job that everyone would know. Next came anger. I'd given 20 years of my life to this company. Finally, I was besieged by a sense of helplessness. *Could I possibly talk my way out of this or was it a fait accompli?*

When you've been in a job for twenty years — and especially one that is so visible — that role becomes inextricably intertwined with your personal identity. It feels like so much more than losing a job.

I could have easily let my anger at the ABC execs take me by the neck and strangle me. I could have also let my fear of future unemployment totally paralyze me.

But somehow a cooler head prevailed and rather than worry about what the future might bring, and whether it would be as good, I thankfully focused on how I should handle myself during this pivotal point in my life, because I was going to have to do it in front of America. I decided that I would not vent or question the ABC execs' decision publicly and that I would leave the show with grace and dignity. Make no mistake, I was devastated. I was hurt. I'd given the network my loyalty, to say nothing of the lost sleep my pre-dawn wakeups cost me. But I made a decision to keep those feelings private. Sure, I vented to my close friends, but I never gave one negative interview, and I've never regretted making that choice.

I can hardly believe it myself that I never sought revenge. I guess living a good life and being happy and successful is a kind of a sweet revenge in and of itself.

I finally decided that the sun would come up tomorrow, even without GMA.

Leaving GMA also meant that my connection with our viewers was being taken away from me. It would be years later, when Facebook came about, that I would finally get the chance to reconnect with many of those morning friends.

Why do we all seem to be so resistant to change in our lives? I think it's because we all fear the unknown! That's certainly what I was concerned about. I had no idea what would come next.

Think about it. How many of you were

afraid of the dark when you were little? Come on, weren't most of us a tiny bit scared? Why? Because you couldn't see what was there. The dark made us edgy and uncomfortable. Our minds played all sorts of tricks on us as we thought about what might be lurking in that shadow or in that corner of the closet we couldn't quite see. We are only born with two fears — the fear of falling and the fear of loud noises. Every other fear is learned, which means it can be overcome.

As adults, changes in life can often mimic those dark corners and thus can bring on some of those same feelings of uncertainty. What's out there that might make us uncomfortable? Wouldn't it be so much easier if we could just turn on the lights and take a peek?

Psychologists tell us that the first step to managing the fear of change is to look at how we are presenting the change to ourselves. They say we should try imagining the change as wonderful and exciting and see ourselves moving forward with ease and not focus so much on what might be different or missing in our life. For instance, many people who have to give up driving at a certain age feel angry and helpless. But in today's world, they can discover Uber, Lyft, or even a service like Go Go Grandparents, all transportation services where they can instantly have someone else driving them where they need to go, and they don't have to get behind the wheel or stew over traffic. Plus, they have company along the way. Of course, it's difficult when life throws us a curve and we're required to find a new course, but we can eliminate a lot of stress from that challenge by letting go of disappointment or fear and forging a new path.

"In life we cannot avoid change, we cannot avoid loss. Freedom and happiness are found in the flexibility and ease with which we move through change."
— SIDDHARTHA GAUTAMA

Ironically, one of the first opportunities that came my way after leaving *Good Morning America* was a request from American Express to be the keynote speaker at a huge international travel conference in Edinburgh, Scotland. I guess I have to tell you why that's ironic.

I had a fear of public speaking.

Yep, I'm not kidding. Despite an audience of 20 million viewers a week on television, the mere thought of speaking in front of several hundred people in a live situation had always unnerved me. And I'm not just talking butterflies in my stomach here; I am talking about full-blown, red, blotchy hives on my chest! I know, after working on television all those years, it seems pretty odd. How could I be nervous in front of a few hundred people when millions of people saw me every day? Well, guess what? I didn't see any of them!

For many years, I avoided public speaking at all costs. It was always easy to turn down a speech while I was hosting a live morning show. I could never predict what would be happening in the world so how could I possibly commit to being at an organization's event? Good excuse, right?

The event in Scotland was just what I needed to start letting go of my long-time fear of public speaking. While I can barely even remember walking onto that stage in Edinburgh that first time, I did it. And you know what? It was exciting! Scary, but exciting. Suddenly, I was determined to let go of my unwarranted fear so that I could accept other speaking opportunities. I saw an exciting future that could be mine, but only if I could release the fear.

A few months later, renowned motivational speaker Tony Robbins asked me to join him on his national speaking tour. Joining Tony's tour meant I would be giving 26 speeches in the first year, talking in front of audiences of 24,000 attendees or more. It was a daunting challenge, but clearly an opportunity to begin reinventing myself. However, I still wondered, *Even with the guru of inspirational speaking, would I be able to do it? Would I have the power to change my life?*

You know that saying, "You can't teach an old dog new tricks"? Well I'm here to tell you, oh yes, you can!

> "When life puts you in tough
> situations, don't say Why me? . . .
> say Why not me?"
> — UNKNOWN

Today I average over twenty speeches a year. I travel around the country sharing my experiences with audiences of all ages. It is arguably one of the most rewarding and enjoyable parts of my career. I almost can't even believe it; it's such a dramatic turn-around.

In the beginning, I had been uneasy about writing my speeches, fearing that I'd have nothing poignant to say. Okay, so I've obviously let go of that fear.

Now, just try to stop me from writing. I think it's fair to say that I am a true example of someone who has abandoned her fear and survived! I have turned that angst into a complete and joyful passion. I encourage you to embrace change in your life too; it may pleasantly surprise you.

"To each of us, at certain points of our lives, there come opportunities to rearrange our formulas and assumptions — not necessarily to be rid of the old, but more to profit from adding something new."
— LEO BUSCAGLIA

CHAPTER 20
WHEN THERE ARE
LUMPS IN THE ROAD

"Few journeys through life are
uninterrupted. Take these pauses
as a time to reflect, refresh and
recharge and they cease to be
perceived as interruptions."
— JIM PHILLIPS

I saw a poster in a doctor's office the other day that I loved. It read, *When life's road has potholes and speed bumps, it makes you a better driver.* It doesn't always feel like that when we hit a bump, but I usually find that my perspective changes when I'm a few miles down the road looking back.

For some of us, those bumps come in the form of lumps, literally, and we are challenged to go into high gear and fight for our lives. That is what happened to me when I was diagnosed with breast cancer. You've heard me talk about this before, but I mention it again in this book because the most significant risk factors for this type of cancer are (1) being female and (2) aging. Roughly 95 percent of all breast cancers in the U.S. occur in women aged 40 and older. The good news is that the largest group of cancer survivors happens to be breast cancer survivors. We are more than 2.9 million strong, and a lot of that has to ultimately do with how we care for ourselves mentally and emotionally, as well as physically, once we find out.

In general, aging can bring unwelcome diagnoses — many of which are curable or at least manageable given today's medical advances. Learning how to cope with difficult news in the health realm takes fortitude, but hey, we survived this long. We must be loaded with fortitude, right? I know I discovered unknown sources of it in myself during my battle with cancer.

When I heard those words, "You have breast cancer," my life came to a screeching halt. My first lesson in the challenging fight for my life was that cancer did not care about any of my plans. I had always assumed that breast cancer was something that would happen to some other woman, not to me. But now here I was hearing the unimaginable.

I had gotten a 3D mammogram that day,

which was negative, but in the ultrasound that followed, I learned I had an aggressive form of breast cancer called Triple Negative. It was a fluke that I even had that ultrasound. It was only because a few years earlier I'd interviewed breast cancer expert Dr. Susan Love about mammogram screenings. I told Dr. Love I found them nervewracking because I was always called back for more pictures, although the technicians said it was only because I had dense breasts, so it was hard to see much. With that, Dr. Love said I should be having regular ultrasounds in addition to mammograms. It turns out that her advice very likely saved my life.

It's not easy telling people that you have cancer, or any other serious disease for that matter. For me, it felt like I was flawed, no longer a healthy vibrant individual. I remember sitting in the salon the day I got my head shaved. I wanted to feel like GI Joan but when I looked in the mirror, no getting around it, I looked like a cancer patient.

With some reservation at the outset, I decided to go public with my diagnosis in the hopes that it might give me the opportunity to make an important impact on women's health. You know that saying, "The truth will set you free"? Well, that was certainly the case for me. As soon as I took my story wide, the breast cancer community reached out to me to speak around the country. I began documenting and sharing my cancer battle online. I finally felt like I was becoming a real warrior in my battle. This public campaign shifted my mental focus from *my own personal cancer* to *the fight against all cancer.*

It's been said that helping others helps yourself. This was certainly true for me. My advocacy changed my breast cancer journey in the most positive way and my life was starting to take on a whole new purpose. As I was battling my cancer, I was helping others. I once read that when you overcome loss, you gain new strength. I just hoped I was as strong as everyone kept saying I was.

> "A woman is like a tea bag, you can't tell how strong she is until you put her in hot water.
> — ELEANOR ROOSEVELT

I traveled the country sharing what I'd learned on my journey. I went to Washington, D.C., and knocked on senators' doors to lobby for needed changes in health care policy. I had found a new community, the breast cancer community, and I was awe-struck by the power and sense of loyalty that this unique sorority had. No matter where I went, whether to a conference, a breast cancer awareness luncheon, or to a Pink Run/Walk, it seemed that every female member was instinctually reaching out and checking on other women there, lending their advice or simply their strength. Those wonderful women made me a better person. They taught me to more fully give of myself. They instilled in me a deeper, resounding compassion for each and every woman who walks our path. They made me more resilient. They helped me to believe I would beat my cancer, that I would make it over the finish line. And I did. I'm happy to report that after sixteen rounds of aggressive chemo, as well as surgery and six weeks of radiation, I remain cancer free.

> "Cancer didn't bring me to my knees. It brought me to my feet."
> — MICHAEL DOUGLAS

Help Yourself by Helping Others

As I've connected with a lot of women around the country in recent years, I've repeatedly heard how confusing they find the conflicting reports about how to care for your breast health. Top of that list, for many women, is when to get a mammogram. This has become my bully pulpit of sorts, so please indulge me. The thoughts I share here may be lifesaving information for any one of you.

There have been a lot of news stories about recently relaxed mammogram guidelines that suggest women should delay the start of mammograms until age 45 or even 50. Frankly, nothing infuriates me more.

I often hear from women in their early forties, and even younger, who are being diagnosed with breast cancer. If those 40-something-year-old women had followed the new guidelines, I shudder to think about what might have happened to them in the intervening years.

There is no debate on this issue in my mind. I can't stress enough how important it is for women to get their mammograms annually beginning at age 40.

Mammograms are the best diagnostic tool we have right now for finding breast cancer as early as possible, so every woman must be sure to get her screenings. It is also imperative that we ask our referring doctor or our radiology lab about our breast density when we have our mammograms.

When we are young, our breast tissue

tends to be quite dense. As most women age, that dense tissue is replaced by fatty tissue. Cancer can be detected more readily during a mammogram in women with fatty tissue. However, that is not the case for all women.

About half of the women in this country still have dense breast tissue well into their 40s, 50s, and beyond. For us, breast cancer is not easy to see on a mammogram. Dense, fibrous tissue shows up as white on a mammogram as does cancer. All too often that means the cancer is hard to discern. It's like looking for a snowball in a snowstorm. For those women — women like me — an ancillary test is required. This is usually an ultrasound, also called a sonogram. Current statistics indicate that if a woman is diagnosed with one of the common breast cancers today, it's caught at an early stage, and is located only in the breast, she has a 99 percent chance of survival. So you can see that early vigilance and asking questions can make all the difference in the world.

My lump in the road greatly challenged me, but it also steered me onto a new path in my life for which I am most grateful. For me, my cancer survival meant a new beginning.

"You are here to find your gift — perfect it — and give something back."

— DAVID VISCOTT,
AUTHOR OF *EMOTIONAL RESILIENCE*

It hardly seems possible as I sit here writing today that I ever heard the dreaded words, "You have cancer." It took a year out of my life. Now, though, I can see the bigger picture: That it is a fight we wage and hopefully one we win before we get on with living the rest of our lives, looking at our battle at a distance well behind us. But when you are in the middle of cancer treatment, it's almost impossible to see it from that perspective. That's why I need to continue to stand as a symbol of hope for all those women who are still waging their battle. I cannot leave this post.

As someone in the public eye, I have often felt the need to use my platform to spread this message. But the truth is that a number of us will hit bumps in the road as we age. Hopefully they will be less severe than mine. When and if that happens, it helps to become beacons of hope for the others around us, no matter how well known or anonymous we may believe ourselves to be. The women who inspired me at the various breast cancer awareness and support events

I spoke of earlier certainly weren't celebrities, but they created their own platforms and bore the responsibility to model strength and spread information as well, if not better, than most celebs. With adversity, almost more than with age, comes the wisdom that unity, perseverance, and purpose really matter.

"My expiration date just got extended, so with the precious time I have left, I try to live consciously and righteously and leave this planet a better place than it was before I got here."
— MARISA MARCHETTO, CARTOONIST AND BESTSELLING AUTHOR

CHAPTER 21
DECLINE TO DECLINE

> "Of all the self-fulfilling prophecies
> in our culture, the assumption that
> aging means decline and poor health
> is probably the deadliest."
> — MARILYN FERGUSON

I've always admired my husband's grand-mother Rose, who everyone quite appropriately called Rosie because she had an uncanny ability to let things roll off her back and remain positive and grateful for the wonderful life she had. Rosie always appeared to be in control of her outlook and never seemed to let anything get her down.

At the age of 90, Rosie went to the hospital for a minor procedure but ended up staying for a week and having double bypass surgery. Once back home, we got word that Rosie was not doing well in her recovery, that she just didn't seem to be bouncing back. How could that be?

That didn't sound like our Rosie!

My husband and I flew to Fort Lauderdale, Florida, along with his parents, to see what we could do to lift Rosie's spirits. As we entered her home, I immediately noticed it was dark and gloomy. All the drapes and blinds were closed, the lights were dim, and Rosie was curled up in her recliner with several throws draped over her.

Waking Up Rosie!

We immediately pulled back all the drapes and opened up all the glass sliding doors, letting in the brilliant Florida sunshine along with some fresh air. Phew! It was almost as if we'd given her a whopping shot of vitamin B12. Rosie began peeling off the layers of blankets that had been covering her and sat up in her chair. When I looked over at her, I saw a smile start to appear. What a difference that simple change in her environment had made on her brain and her attitude toward the day!

Now we were on a roll. We were sprinkling enthusiasm around the house like it was fairy dust and it was working its magic. We were determined to change Rosie's outlook and bring back her love of life. She was not ready to check out at all! I discovered she liked milkshakes, so I jumped in the car and hunted for a Wendy's. When I reappeared with a chocolate Frosty (her favorite), she seemed almost childlike. It was a small gesture, but it reminded her of the simple joys in life.

Before long she was animated again and telling amusing stories about the old days. We were all laughing and making plans for a family reunion. These seemingly tiny steps had made such an enormous impact on her mindset and thus her health. It worked!

We had given Rosie the jump-start that she needed. It wasn't long before she made a complete recovery and was her usual upbeat self again, proudly telling everyone her age and adding that she didn't even need glasses to read or put on her makeup. Rosie always called to mind something Mark Twain once said, "Age is an issue of mind over matter. If you don't mind, it doesn't matter."

Some people dread the idea of birthdays or of getting older; however, Rosie always said that they were wonderful reminders of the breadth of love and joy that she had been able to experience in life.

Never Let a Stumble Be the End of the Journey

Ten years after that double bypass surgery, we were all planning Rosie's 100th birthday party. She still dressed to the nines every single day, always wearing bright colors and paying close attention to her jewelry, makeup, and hairstyle. Her hands may have been a little shaky, but she still applied her own make-up, and she insisted on her favorite brands of moisturizer, face powder, and green eyeshadow. And believe me, family members ran out to replenish her supplies of it because deep down everyone hoped we would care as much about ourselves as she did when we got to be her age.

Rosie's ability to remain positive and happy about aging — in fact, to be downright grateful for it — taught us all an important life lesson. It is our choice how we approach our advanced years, how we face birthdays, how we deal with the aches and pains of our aging bodies, and whether we choose gratitude for a life well lived.

Personally, I want to be just like Rosie when I grow up.

"We should start referring to 'age' as 'levels,' so when you're at LVL 80, it

363

sounds more Badass than just being an old person."

— UNKNOWN

Rosie always reminded me of my mom since she, too, had that uncanny ability to let life's troubles roll off her back. Ironically, my mother used to tell me to always look at my life through rose-colored glasses.

Those must have been the glasses I had on the day I went to help rescue Rosie!

Mom also used to tell me that one of the best ways to keep our lives exciting and worth living was to always have plans, lots of them. She said making interesting plans for the future allow us to have something to look forward to.

Another of my mom's vintage mottos was, *Half the fun of doing anything is anticipating and planning for it,* so she would throw a party or take a trip once a year, and she clearly reveled in the anticipation.

Over the years, I have found that having plans and goals has helped me to keep excited and moving forward. Thanks, Mom aren't our moms always right?

This concept of planning for an exciting future is perhaps one of the best-kept secrets of successful aging. Conversely, assuming that our future will be one of decline is downright dangerous.

When people assume they'll deteriorate as they age, they do, in fact, decline. I first encountered this notion in an article about Deepak Chopra's bestselling book *Ageless Body, Timeless Mind.* I recall reading the words, "People don't grow old. People get old when they stop growing," and thinking to myself, *Well, he sure is an optimist!* Then of course, I immediately went out and bought a copy of the book.

Chopra really made me think about the concept of aging and of being old. He suggests that we have greater control over our own vitality than we realize. In fact — and I'm paraphrasing here — we may be responsible for draining the energy from our own lives by the very expectations and beliefs we carry. For example, if we anticipate being useless, we will certainly trigger the physical, mental, and emotional changes that render us that way!

Although it appeals to common sense that we grow old because we simply wear out, no wear-and-tear theory of aging has actually held up under close scrutiny.

The concept that most amazed me in the book was when Chopra suggested that aging is "something your body has largely *learned* to do." He explains that we program our minds quite unconsciously. We have fed it ideas and assumptions for years we don't even know we hold to be true. What an eye-opener!

Behavioral psychologists have estimated that just the verbal cues we picked up from our parents in early childhood still run inside our heads all these years later. Given how many times they've been said, heard, and then replayed by us, we can assume we've been under roughly 25,000 hours of conditioning. This conditioning has created the expectation that we will decline, and so we do. Think back to that resilient and persevering Bedouin tribeswoman I spoke about earlier in this book — the one who had no concept of age. She was clearly *not* fed the same concepts about aging as we were!

According to Deepak Chopra, there are three ways that we can measure our age: chronologically, biologically, and psychologically. Would it surprise you to discover — especially after considering the example of that tribeswoman — that the most unreliable gauge of the three is chronological?

Regular physical exercise and better lifestyle choices can reverse the effects of biological aging, including high blood pressure, excess body fat, and decreased muscle mass, among others. And a positive psychological outlook can certainly turn back the hands of time.

Chopra tells us that if we live a lifestyle that involves listening to others attentively, giving them our time and respect, co-operating with them, and doing things for reasons other than furthering our own needs, we will age well.

I'm a total Deepak Chopra devotee, but even if you don't follow his writing the way I do, you must agree that his perspective here is empowering, right? After reading Chopra's book I changed my approach to aging completely. I no longer perceive it as a threat to my many desirable goals. I now think of my later years as something to get excited about and plan for. Holy moly, what a difference it's made!

"The greatest discovery of my generation is that a human being can change his life by changing his attitude of mind."
— WILLIAM JAMES

I think we all know what it means to create a bucket list. For many people, it's a list of countries they'd like to visit and explore. Others might want to pursue an unfulfilled dream. For my mother-in-law, Janey

Konigsberg, it was getting her college diploma. In the 1950s, Janey had been a senior in college when she got married and became pregnant with her first child. Times were very different then, and as soon as her baby belly began to show, the university insisted that she leave school, two months shy of her graduation. She had always planned to go back and get that diploma, but three more children by the age of 25 changed those plans. For Janey's 70th birthday, her daughters arranged with the university for Janey to finally graduate. An English major, she was given one last assignment: to write a paper about how life had changed for women since she left college. Janey had loads of fun with that assignment, and we had fun cheering her on as she walked across that stage in her cap and gown at 70 to finally get her diploma. That's a big one to check off a bucket list!

While traditional bucket lists are fun, I'm going to suggest that we create another kind of bucket list — one more like a checklist of objectives to pursue in our future. Think of it as a blueprint for how we want to live our lives going forward — or, as others like to say, as we age.

To help create this list ask yourself the question, "What are you doing with the rest of your life?" Hey, wait, isn't that the title of a song? Or a cheesy pick-up line from the 70s?

To design a happiness plan, it helps to paint a picture of our future life doing things that bring us joy. Once we create this vision plan, it will help guide us toward achieving that life.

Here are some questions to help provide greater detail to the plan:

- Do I see myself travelling and soaking up the history of faraway places?
- Am I more of a homebody who prefers to live close to a golf course so I can work on my game every day?
- Would I enjoy setting up an art studio in my home? Or perhaps planting a vegetable and herb garden? Would following that with cooking classes make life even more robust?
- Do I want to spend more quality time with my grown children and grandchildren? (I guess you should confer with them on this one. LOL.)
- Do I look forward to having lots of leisure time and to socializing with my friends, playing cards, and going to dinner or to the movies?
- Do I see myself attending lectures,

plays, or concerts at a nearby college, learning new things and mingling with young, intellectually curious students?

- Do I want to live somewhere that will allow me to spend more time in nature, taking walks or even hikes? Maybe living by a lake is in my future.
- What can I do that will keep me laughing?
- What have I always wanted to do that I never had time to try before?

These are all questions that can help us design a life for ourselves which will keep us happy, socially connected, and content. These are important plans — plans my mom would surely approve of!

I seriously recommend you take me up on this challenge and start your own list! Are you married? If so, it's a good idea to ask your spouse to join you in creating this game plan for the future, just to make sure that you're both on the same page. In fact, this exercise — planning a fun future for the two of you — just might add a little spark to your marriage.

So what kind of plans would we find on your list? Do you have a secret hidden hobby or passion? Are you an ace at pool or badminton? What about bowling? I hear pickleball is becoming popular! This is our chance to be a kid again. Give yourself permission to play!

There's no right way to create your list, and if you're evolving as I suspect you are, that list will very likely change over time too. Climbing Mt. Kilimanjaro has remained on my bucket list for years, much to my husband's dismay. But as I've aged, my list has morphed, and that serious climb up the highest peak in Africa has been replaced by a desire to take a photojournalism trip through the Serengeti reserve on the same continent. The only *climbing* that adventure involves is ambling up into a jeep before focusing my lens.

> "Make today so awesome that yesterday gets jealous."
> — UNKNOWN

I'm also looking forward to unapologetically curling up with a good book. The prospect of being able to read as much as I want, and never feel like I'm neglecting some other pressing responsibility in my life, is incredibly tantalizing to me.

Life is all about the choices we make for ourselves. Some people, as they get older, just sit back and let things take their course, while others choose to find engaging pursuits brimming with stimulation, excitement, joy, and happiness. Which group do you think will help you stay young at heart and filled with laughter and enthusiasm? I know, this was an easy one to answer.

> "As soon as you feel too old to do a thing, DO IT."
> — MARGARET DELAND, AMERICAN AUTHOR

It's up to us to keep our fire burning and to retain our love of life. Happiness can be found all around us, but we have to open our eyes and our heart. Here are my ten favorite ways to stay happy and *decline to decline.*

Get Some Sunshine and Fresh Air: As my mom got older, she used to joke that "her get up and go, got up and went." Yet even when she was in her 90s, Mom still loved going for walks outside in the bright light of day. Research suggests that light stimulates the brain chemicals that improve our mood. They especially recommend getting that sunlight first thing in the morning, when it can give us an extra energy boost.

Put More Energy into Your Voice: Before

you tell me I'm nuts, haven't you ever noticed how some people start talking more softly as they age. Don't let that happen. In fact, put on some music and sing. You never know, it might even entice you to get up and dance. *That* could put a spring in your step!

Tackle a Task: Call me crazy but crossing things off my to-do list can always give me a sense of calm and cheer, especially if it's making that long-postponed doctor appointment or filling out those pesky insurance forms. Getting stuff done — even the mundane things — greatly contributes to our inner peace.

My daughter Lindsay, who is a busy mom of two little ones and also vice president of my production company, offered a highlighting trick for those days that seem to slip away before anything gets crossed off our to-do list. She suggested that we look at our list each morning and highlight 2 to 3 items. Those things are non-negotiable. Those are TODAY tasks. It could be answering an annoying but necessary email or booking a flight. But those tasks must get done before the day is over. Prioritizing like this is a wonder!

Lindsay also uses a notebook where she

keeps daily reminders, so she never loses a name, number, or important piece of information. She has found that if she changes the color pen she uses from day to day, she can see the progression of things as well as the things that have remained undone for a week. She'll also notice the new things that were added each day. As she says, "It's also an excuse to buy pretty colored pens. Let's be honest, I came up with this idea in the aisle at Staples."

Reach Out: Keeping close bonds with other people is one of the most important keys to happiness. Take a moment to send a card or an email or to make a call to a friend you haven't seen in a while.

Do a Good Deed: Making other people happy is a sure-fire way to make yourself happy. Take a moment to pass along a compliment, a thank you, or maybe just some useful information that will help someone. If you're creative, you could make a photo album for a friend or family member, bake something for a neighbor, or crochet a blanket for a baby. Whaaat? You think I'm getting carried away?

Act Happy: *Duh!* Sorry, but that's what

my kids would say. I know it may seem like a silly suggestion, but research shows that even an artificially induced smile can actually boost our mood. Plus, if we're smiling, then other people perceive us as being happier and friendlier and, well, you see where I'm going with this.

Watch a Funny TV Show or Movie: I happen to love movies whether they're funny, action-packed, or documentaries. Experts have measured people's responses to watching funny movies and TV shows and found that laughter approximates a mood-lifting drug, except with no side effects. And in my book, having a good ol' belly laugh can almost be considered an aerobic activity.

Learn Something New: The good news is that in today's world we can search the Internet and discover just about anything. Then again, we can go to a bookstore and buy a book about it. I love bookstores. I'm out of control there. I usually walk out with an armful of good reads. According to the experts, we just need to make sure we pick a topic that really interests us, and not something we think we *should* or *need to* learn about.

Follow a Passion: When my husband's Aunt Millie was 91, she lost her husband and was overwhelmed with sadness. Her family encouraged her to take up painting, which had been a passion of hers in her younger years. She literally came alive with her newfound endeavor and it wasn't long before her apartment resembled an art gallery. Everyone in the family was thrilled to see Millie get her life back, and we all have her works hanging in our homes.

Reconnect with Your Inner Child: The stories of Aunt Millie continue. For many years my husband would hold a massive family reunion at one of the summer camps he owns and runs in Maine. It was tradition during these gatherings for everyone to play in the family baseball game. And I do mean *everyone.* Well, when it was Aunt Millie's turn to be up at bat, she exclaimed to the family that she could still swing and that she only needed someone to run the bases for her. And yep, you guessed it: 94-year-old Millie got a base hit! Millie didn't want to stand on the sidelines and watch, she wanted to be on the winning team. Oh my, the power of play! I want to be able to hit and round first base when I am Millie's age! LOL!

Aunt Millie taught me that it doesn't matter if you run around the bases slowly; it only matters that you continue to get up to bat. I'm like her; I don't want to retire to the sidelines. I want to stay in the game. How about you? I say we all decide to *decline to decline* and walk forward into our later years with an expectation that we are going to age the way they do in the big leagues — still full of fire and determination.

For once in my life I'm going to obey what my mother told me to do: I'm going to keep making plans. Lots of them. Our mothers are always right, aren't they? That's what I tell my kids!

I know one thing for sure. When I get old, I don't want people thinking "What a sweet little old lady that Joan Lunden is."

I want them saying, "Oh crap, what's she up to now?"

Chapter 22
Friends Are Therapists
You Can Drink With

"A good friend knows all your stories.
A best friend helped you write them."
— Unknown

Are you ever jealous of your children? I'm serious. Because I sure am. I mean it. What really makes me yearn to have what they have is the number of really good friends in their lives. This holds true for all three of my older daughters — Jamie, Lindsay, and Sarah. Each of them enjoys a cadre of besties collected from high school, summer camp, college, and their careers. I don't know how they find the time to see them all socially, but somehow, they do.

"Friends are the family we
choose for ourselves."
— Edna Buchanan

When I take a mental inventory, adding up people from my high school, college, and summer camp days — even using both hands and carrying the one — the sad truth is, I don't have that many really close friends from those chapters in my life. Maybe it's because I didn't linger and savor those days enough. Candidly, I skipped a grade and couldn't wait to graduate from high school. I was too eager to set off to see the world. It's not that I didn't have friendships back then. I did. But I had ambition and big dreams. I had wanderlust. I didn't go back home to visit much so I lost touch with the friends I had.

The same holds true for my college days. I didn't follow the normal path and attend one college for four years, living in close quarters among peers in dorms where lifelong friendships are fostered. Instead, I spent my first semester in a rather unique setting, travelling around the globe through a program called World Campus Afloat. Today this floating college is called Semester at Sea. Although I formed friendships while visiting more than a dozen countries, the students on board with me returned to their respective universities throughout the U.S. when our semester together ended.

It was the most amazing introduction to the world. I was hooked on the adrenaline that came from travelling to new and exciting places. The following semester I moved to Mexico City where I attended a university called Universidad de Las Americas. I made friendships there; however, this was also a study-abroad campus where most students attended for only one or two semesters rather than for four years, as one does on a traditional university campus. Two more colleges would follow — a little time spent here, a little time there — all exciting, but I never hunkered down long enough to create lasting bonds like the ones my daughters enjoy.

It wasn't until I moved to New York City and entered the work world that I laid down roots and started forming enduring friendships I still hold dear today. My closest friends are the women I've worked with on various shows, books, and media campaigns. In particular, they are the women who worked with me at *Good Morning America* and travelled the world with me, running my office and many aspects of my life. They may have started out as my personal assistants, but over the years we have shared one another's joys and sorrows and have always turned to one another for support and advice. They have truly become sisters to me. When something uplifting occurs, I can't wait to tell them, and when I'm troubled by something, they are my first call. They provide a hearty laugh, a shoulder to cry on, and a warm embrace, depending upon the situation. I feel that they always bring out the best in me and help me to believe in myself. And I hope I do the same for them.

> "The most called upon prerequisite of a friend, is an accessible ear."
> — MAYA ANGELOU

When I get together with girlfriends, a quick lunch always seems to last for three hours. A magical feeling takes over when I'm with my close friends. There is a sense of freedom and safety that comes with loyal camaraderie that allows us to talk about almost anything without fear of judgement. We can giggle and laugh hard, which is so good for the soul, and in fact, for our immune system. I think we would all agree that when we are together it's like time hasn't passed. We walk away not only feeling happier, but I would say even a bit younger. I have come to believe that friendships are truly the fountain of youth. We must nurture them.

The Positive Power of Social Connections

Research shows that people with strong social networks who spend quality time with friends and family are more likely to live longer than people who are lonely. Social connections are one of the leading predictors of successful aging.

According to the Harvard Study of Adult Development, the relationships we cultivate and maintain in our lives have a more important impact on aging than the events we experience. They are associated with a 50 percent reduced risk of early death. *Wow.*

Loneliness exacts a grave toll; it is said to be comparable to the risk of smoking up to 15 cigarettes a day! It exceeds the risk of alcohol consumption, and it exceeds the risk of physical inactivity, obesity, and even the risk of air pollution.

There is nothing that will accelerate decline more than isolation. What's more, loneliness seems to pose the greatest risk for elderly people who are also prone to depression.

Gerontologists studying the power of connection have found that people who go to a religious service regularly tend to live 2 to 3 years longer than people who do not go to services regularly. It doesn't seem to matter what religion the services are centered around, just that the person goes frequently, for when people are part of a community, they have a greater sense of belonging and tend to have more emotional support.

If you haven't accumulated an abundance of friendships throughout your life, it's *never* too late to start! Sometimes friends made later in life are the best kind because they tend to be at the same stage of life and share many of our current interests.

So *right now,* make a plan to go somewhere you are likely to find others with common interests. It could be a church group, a book or travel club, an art class, a gym or Zumba class, a library reading or lecture — anywhere you might meet likeminded people. And don't be shy. Make a point of introducing yourself, start a conversation, and nurture a new friendship. No matter your age, these kinds of exchanges could lead to new and uplifting bonds in life.

"Count your age by friends, not years.
Count your life by smiles, not tears."
— JOHN LENNON

CHAPTER 23
AN ATTITUDE OF GRATITUDE

"Why are people afraid of getting older?
You feel wiser. You feel more mature. You
feel like you know yourself better. You
would trade that for softer skin? Not me!"
— ANNA KOURNIKOVA,
PROFESSIONAL TENNIS PLAYER

We've all heard the phrase, *As you grow
older, you grow wiser.* It may sound like
something people say to appease us, but
seriously, we really do grow wiser! I no
longer feel the need to rush through life as
though I'm a participant on *The Amazing
Race.* And because I'm not hurrying this
way and that, I also feel as if I have a better
perspective on my world. I'm more relaxed
with who I am and more grateful for everything that I have. I don't give much credence
to thoughts about what might still be missing. Granted, I've always been a glass-half-
full kind of person, but the vantage point

age now lends me seems to leave me happier and more serene.

When we are making our way in the world, starting careers in our 20s, families in our 30s, and new ventures in our 40s and 50s, we tend to wake up thinking about all the things we need to do in order to get all the things we want to have. And we maintain that focus all day long.

I now find myself in my 60s waking up thinking about how grateful I am for the life I've lived and the people I'm surrounded by. Gratitude helps us notice the good things in our lives, and that helps us experience positive feelings, not only about ourselves but about our world in general.

"Cherish all your happy moments;
They make a fine cushion for old age."
— BOOTH TARKINGTON

The simple act of counting our blessings is a powerful tool. It helps us maintain a positive attitude. An appreciative person is able to move through life with a better immune system, fewer ulcers, lower blood pressure, less stress, and more laughter and less illness. Sounds like a pretty good plan to me!

"Happiness is not how much you have.
Happiness is how much you appreciate
what you have."
— JAMIE KRAUSS HESS

Gratitude is actually one of the best researched emotions because it may be the most powerful one. The study of gratitude has found that it isn't just a state of mind; it's inextricably linked to the function of the brain and body. Gratitude activates the parasympathetic nervous system (the relaxing part of that system), whereas negative emotions activate the sympathetic nervous system (the part that triggers the fight-or-flight response we spoke of earlier). The many positive effects of gratitude include lowering our blood pressure, increasing relaxation, and promoting better rest, not only making it easier to fall asleep but also to stay asleep longer!

Studies have also found that a strong sense of gratitude helps to reduce the stress hormone cortisol and increase the hormone DHEA, which promotes a more tranquil state. In the end, it's also believed to strengthen our immune system by increasing the level of immunoglobulin A, an antibody that is one of our body's first lines of defense against viruses. In short, something as simple as gratitude can lead to a longer, healthier life.

"Getting old is like climbing a mountain;
you get a little out of breath, but the view
is much better!"
— INGRID BERGMAN

An important part of finding gratitude in our life, of course, is coming to an acceptance of some things as they are. I think we all intellectually understand that it's better for us to stop resisting that which we cannot change and move on, but in some ironic way, that's a truth that is often difficult to *accept* too.

The point is that acceptance is a choice — a trying one, no doubt, but a choice, nevertheless. Many people go through life seeing things how they want them to be, instead of seeing them as they are. But just because we may want things to be different, doesn't mean they will be. Sometimes — not always, but sometimes — we need to embrace things as they actually are in order to make life a little easier on ourselves in the long run. I think most of you will agree, that with age, accepting people or situations we can't change becomes a lot less difficult. Maybe we've learned through experience or maybe we just don't give a crap anymore. Sorry, just being honest. But seriously, things that use to get under my skin just roll off my back now.

Of course, if you find it absolutely necessary to close a door and let out a bloodcurdling scream before accepting your circumstance, go right ahead. Just bear in mind that, while there may be evidence that screaming out in a moment of frustration or anger lets off steam, screaming can also take a physical toll on the body. I've experienced it. I once went into my bedroom closet to scream out of frustration and could actually *feel* my body react. I decided right then and there that I wouldn't do that again. My health is more important. It likely raised my blood pressure. And what's worse is that the outburst only gave me a few seconds of relief! Acceptance, on the other hand, can lower your blood pressure *and* last a lifetime.

"The road to happiness is always under construction."
— BRIAN LUKE SEAWARD, PH.D.

Once you try it, if you haven't already, I'm sure you'll find acceptance and gratitude to be incredibly freeing feelings. When

I was going through a divorce, it seemed like every call with my ex would spiral into a fight. There was so much emotion involved that the dumbest little remark could make things flair up. Then one day when the phone rang, I decided that this pattern had to stop. It was negatively impacting my happiness and my physical well-being. I couldn't imagine why I was allowing it to continue. Before picking up the receiver I decided this call would not be the same.

Frankly, I think that call was one of the most important of my life. After a very civil, non-emotional exchange, I hung up and never looked back. That's the day that I learned acceptance is a choice. And it's a good one in my book.

We are all going to experience complex emotional situations and confrontations in our lives, so it's important to remember that acceptance can safeguard us from falling down that rabbit hole.

"Life's a journey — travel light."
— UNKNOWN

To keep things light while travelling on your journey, I want to share with you a list of ways to cope with life's stresses that a girlfriend sent to me years ago. Ever since I received it, I've kept it in my desk drawer. And whenever I reread it, I laugh just as hard as I did the first time. It's a sure-fire way to bring out the happy in me. I think it will do the same for you as well.

- Accept that some days you're the pigeon, and some days you're the statue.
- Always read stuff that will make you look good if you die in the middle of it.
- Drive carefully. It's not only cars that can be recalled by their maker.
- If you can't be kind, at least have the decency to be vague.
- Never put both feet in your mouth at the same time, because then you won't have a leg to stand on.
- Nobody cares if you can't dance well. Just get up and dance.
- Since it's the early worm that gets eaten by the bird, sleep late.
- The second mouse gets the cheese.
- When everything's coming your way, you're in the wrong lane.
- Birthdays are good for you. The more you have, the longer you live.
- Some mistakes are too much fun to only make once.

- A truly happy person is one who can enjoy the scenery on a detour.
- We could learn a lot from crayons. Some are sharp, some are pretty, and some are dull. Some have weird names, and all are different colors, but they all have to live in the same box.

CHAPTER 24
BE THE PERSON YOU WANT
TO HAVE LUNCH WITH

"I look forward to being older.
When what you look like becomes less
an issue and what you are is the point."
— SUSAN SARANDON

As I've grown older, I've found that I've become much more contemplative, and I consider that a good thing. It also means that for the first time in my life I've slowed down enough to have the time to even think that way.

What has probably surprised me the most is that I'm not always reminiscing about my many travels, accomplishments, or awards, but rather, I'm thinking about how I have conducted my life and about the person that I've become.

This kind of self-introspection can really stop you in your tracks. It forces you to take an inventory of your attributes, and, of course, your annoying traits as well. Think about all the times you've sat around with friends and talked about other people. Sure, you said, "She's so nice and thoughtful" about some, but just as likely you've said (or at least thought), "I'm glad she's not here. She's always such a gossip," or "She's so stuck up and full of herself."

So now imagine your friends sitting around chatting about you. Yes, they definitely talk about you sometimes too. What phrases do you suspect they're using when the discussion turns to your personality?

To help you out on this one, just answer the following question: *If we were all forced to wear a warning label, what would yours say?* Kind? Good listener? Quiet? Funny? A prankster? Loyal? Easy to be around? Alpha female? Interrupter? Social climber? Gossiper? Self-obsessed? Or maybe a Debbie Downer?

Okay, so I know what I have to do next. I have to paint some adjectives on my sign. So here goes.

Good conversationalist (that could easily mean "talks too much")

Always listens and adds to conversation (can be an interrupter)

Always perky (I know this also drives some people crazy)

Easy to be around

393

A pleaser

But seriously, am I fun to be with? Am I a good conversationalist? Do I cut people off? My husband might want to answer that last one. Sorry, honey, I'm going to work on that.

Have I always been there for my family and friends? Have I extended myself sufficiently when people needed something? Have I always been kind enough? Compassionate enough? Understanding enough? Would people say that I have been a fair and generous person? Have I indulged in gossip? These are tough but necessary questions to answer.

> "There is no pillow so soft as a clean conscience."
> — FRENCH PROVERB

Now you try. If someone were to talk with me about you over lunch, how would they characterize you? How do you wish they'd describe you?

I think this is an important and helpful exercise for all of us to do. In fact, I wrote this chapter so that I would have to complete this exercise too. Making the list of what people might say was intense. Making a list of what I'd *like* for them to say was easier. The really tough part was contemplating what I'd like to change about myself moving forward.

> "You cannot rewrite yesterday's news, but you can influence what you read tomorrow morning."
>
> — UNKNOWN

Let me start with what I would like to change about myself. Are you ready for it? *I would like to consciously talk less and listen more.* I'm serious. I know, I know, I've made my living talking and asking questions. It should be easy, right? But it's not. Remaining quiet when I've collected so many interesting stories over the years feels impossible sometimes. God knows, I have a lot of really good ones. But that doesn't mean that I need to share them all the time. Sure, I'm a good guest at a cocktail party, but I'm feeling like I want to back it down and simply be a good listener (who knows what new stories I might add to my repertoire!). Being present and hearing other people be interesting is an adventure of its own. Of course, talking less and listening more could be a tough goal since I seem to like to hear myself talk (LOL), but I'm trying.

> "God gave us two eyes,
> two ears and only one mouth.
> Use them in this ratio."
> — UNKNOWN

As for the attributes that I'd like to be known for — and by extension, those I should strive harder to achieve — here goes:

I hope that my friends and family would describe me as a kind, thoughtful, considerate, and generous person. I also wouldn't mind being described as fun and funny. What the heck, a girl can dream.

I hope that my children would describe me as a loving and understanding mom who is fair and is always there to help and guide them. By the way, for the record, I'd also like my children to describe me as calm and patient, but I'm guessing that one may require a little bit of work on my part.

As a professional, I would hope to be described as a loyal, hard worker who is always kind to my colleagues, and as someone who is principled and honest in my work as a journalist. It's important to me that those who look to me to represent their company, their message, or their network, feel that I've given them my all.

As a person, I would hope that I would be described as someone who led my life with grace, dignity, and honor. I'd like to be remembered as someone who rose to impressive heights but remained down to earth.

And finally, I would hope that the "Lady up above" would judge me — oops, I mean *describe* me — as someone who was compassionate and who strove to inspire and advocate for others. I sure hope she knows I'm someone who has gratitude for the wonderful life I live.

You've probably noticed that I love quotes. I am very much inspired by them. I've gathered a few of my favorite sayings that I believe could guide us in being the very best company to those sitting across the table from us. I hope you enjoy them.

Be so busy improving your life that you have no time to criticize others.

Be somebody who makes everybody feel like a somebody.

Listen to others with the intent to understand; not with the intent to reply.

Character is how you treat those who can do nothing for you.

Be the woman that fixes another woman's crown without telling the world it was crooked.

Don't compare your life to others. There's no comparison between the sun and the moon. They shine when it's their time.

Everybody has a chapter they don't read out loud.

Don't forget that you're human. It's okay to have a meltdown. Just don't unpack and live there.

Don't burn bridges. You'll be surprised how many times you have to cross the same river.

A head full of fears has no space for dreams.

Don't focus on how stressed you are; focus on how blessed you are.

Your vibe attracts your tribe.

Stay away from negative people. They have a problem for every solution.

The less you respond to negative people, the more peaceful your life will become.

Happiness held is the seed; happiness shared is the flower.

Each new day is another chance to change your life.

While I really love the list I compiled, there is another list I've always loved too. Before I share it with you, let me tell you about its author. She was someone whom I've always admired and who truly belongs in a book about aging gracefully. I'm talking about Audrey Hepburn. I was lucky enough to interview her, and I can tell you that she is one of the most natural beauties I've ever met.

Growing up I'd always felt that Audrey Hepburn was the epitome of timeless grace. I hoped I could grow old with the same dignified flair, elegance, and style. Most women I know felt the same way. But few have Hepburn's classic features or her trim little figure. And fewer still have the kind of impeccable taste that brought such sophistication to everything she wore.

One of the times I interviewed Ms. Hepburn was when *Good Morning America* was broadcasting live from the Netherlands. That day she looked exactly how I always pictured her. Classy and exquisite, yet understated. Her hair was pulled back tight into a chic knot and she wore ankle length, slim pants with a little sweater set, and ballet flats. She exuded youth, poise, and charm.

She was on our show to talk about one of the many worthy UNICEF projects for which she relentlessly worked. I felt then that part of her timeless beauty and grace was owed to her mindset; the fact that she always had such a giving heart, that she was making a difference in people's lives all over the world, that she remained inspired, and that her life had purpose and thus joy. I'm convinced that much of her ability to age gracefully came from within.

> "Outer beauty attracts,
> But inner beauty captivated."
> — KATE ANGEL

When I think of all that she was able to accomplish in communities on every continent, I am reminded of how her kindhearted spirit serves as a fine example to all of us trying to age gracefully in this new world of ours.

There are many worthwhile causes that

need volunteers, and Audrey Hepburn clearly modeled how we can stay vibrant and youthful by remaining relevant and useful.

"They may forget your name, but they will never forget how you made them feel."

— MAYA ANGELOU

By helping others, we always help ourselves. Making a difference in the lives of those in need is an elixir that promises much more than any bottle of hair dye ever could. Not that I am willing to ever give up my color, mind you. Here is Audrey's list, originally written by Sam Levenson.

AUDREY HEPBURN'S FAVORITE BEAUTY TIPS

- For attractive lips, speak words of kindness.
- For lovely eyes, seek out the good in people.
- For a slim figure, share your food with the hungry.
- For beautiful hair, let a child run his/ her fingers through it once a day.
- For poise, walk with the knowledge that you never walk alone.

Wow! Wouldn't you love to have lunch with *this* woman? But of course, the question at hand is still: *How would you want the person sitting across from Audrey to be describing . . . you?*

This is a long-term project for most of us, as we are all a work in progress. I'll bet even Audrey Hepburn would have agreed with that statement. It just seems as if that was the kind of person she was.

It's your turn now. How would you define yourself to yourself?

I'll wait while you think about the answer.

Also think about how you would like to broaden that description. We should never underestimate the power we possess to change our lives. So often we tend to define ourselves by what we have done in the past and not by what we are currently doing or what we could be doing in the immediate future. Shouldn't we expand who we are to include all the wonderful things we'd like to be? I bet we would be great at a lot of things we never thought we'd be good at if we just tried.

"Your only limitation is the one which you set up in your own mind."
— NAPOLEON HILL

There are a lot of people reinventing themselves and their lives every day. When I think about reinventing myself, there's a saying that comes to mind, "It's never trespassing when we cross our own boundaries." It's a saying I've always loved because it is so liberating.

We are the ones who set our own parameters. But we can break through those self-imposed restrictions at any time by simply deciding to change our mind. I think of it as turning a little switch in my brain from "I can't do that" to "Just watch me try!"

During the last two decades, I've had the opportunity not only to host TV shows but to pursue lots of new things. I've had roles in several movies and prime-time shows; I've spearheaded media campaigns; I've spoken to audiences all over the world; I created a women's summer getaway camp in Maine; I designed several home goods lines including everything from cookware to bedding, which I sold on QVC; and, of course, I've continued writing books.

I am most certainly not done. The more new projects I say yes to, the more I strengthen my courage muscle, the more comfortable I am trying other new things, and the more excited I become about life.

"Courage is like a muscle.
We strengthen it with use."
— RUTH GORDON

It's never too late to write new chapters in our life story. We are each the authors of our own adventure. We get to write what will be on our next page. We hold the pen.

Our story will be determined not so much by what life brings to us, but by the attitude, passion, and perseverance we bring to life.

CHAPTER 25
BE HAPPY;
IT DRIVES PEOPLE CRAZY

"When I get old, I'm not going to be sitting around knitting. I'm going to be clicking my 'Life Alert' button to see how many hot firefighters show up."

— UNKNOWN

Who can listen to Pharrell Williams's song "Happy" without breaking out in a smile? I know I can't. And do you remember Bobby McFerrin's song "Don't Worry, Be Happy"? I've always loved that tune. One of the first lines is, "In every life we have some trouble, but when you worry, you make it double." To me these songs are more than just lyrical; they are philosophical. They may seem simplistic, but they can have a real impact on our mood, particularly on our sense of contentment and pleasure.

The truth is that we can all have happiness in our lives, for happiness is a choice. (Just like acceptance and how we react to

405

stressors is a choice! Are you seeing a theme here?) It may be a hard concept to grasp — that each of us chooses to be happy, sad, angry, or even bored — but psychologists tell us that all human emotions are choices. That, of course, means that we must take responsibility for our feelings *and* for our own happiness. I actually find it empowering to know that we have that much control over our moods and our lives.

> "A smile is a curve that sets
> everything straight."
> — PHYLLIS DILLER

How do we exercise this kind of control over our happiness? One way to begin is by identifying which of our expectations in life are realistic and which are unrealistic.

Sometimes the higher our expectations, the less we are able to appreciate what we have. If we have unrealistically high expectations, we are often disappointed in people, in jobs, or in relationships. If we can set more appropriate ones, then we are seldom disappointed.

Does the following scenario sound familiar? You have a friend who is always late. Every time you meet up for lunch you end up sitting in a restaurant tapping your foot and feeling annoyed or even hurt. You think, *Doesn't she know this bothers me?*

But here's the thing: If her tardiness is habitual, why are you expecting that *this* time will be any different? In fact, it's said that the definition of insanity is doing the same thing over and over and expecting a different result. All you're doing, really, is setting yourself up for a letdown. Instead, recognize that being on time is not her strength. Use the more realistic expectation that she'll be 15 minutes late to your advantage and catch up on your emails or check out that cute purse at the shop next door first. When we have proper expectations, we're not likely to be disappointed.

I've found that in my quiet, more reflective moments, if I'm truly honest and objective with myself, I can identify my unrealistic expectations. For instance, I want to love cycling, but as much as I try, it just hurts my butt too much. I want to lose my craving for Tostitos, but somehow, they seem to end up in my shopping cart. I want my teenaged children to stop rolling their eyes and maybe even spend a precious Saturday night with me now and then! Don't worry, I'm fully aware that this one is an unrealistic expectation.

Once we recognize an expectation as being unrealistic, we can do one of three things:

Meet it.

Forget it.

Or replace it with something more realistic.

But worrying, fretting, and obsessing over a situation never works. As for the *terrible teens* (oh yes, the *terrible twos* have nothing on this phase!), I must recognize that my kids' sometimes less-than-subtle quest for independence is actually healthy and age-appropriate behavior. Of course, it doesn't hurt to practice deep breathing, and repeat the universal parental mantra, "This too shall pass."

"Don't yell at your kids.
Lean in and whisper, it's much scarier."
— CHRISTINE ALGER

My mom always seemed to be so good at letting things roll off her back and keeping a smile on her face. In fact, her friends all called her "Hap," which was short for "Happy." She seemed to have an uncanny ability to keep life in perspective and was always trying to teach me to do the same. I can remember times when I would go to her to discuss a squabble I was having with

408

someone at school and she would calmly remind me of the old adage, "If you can't say something nice, don't say anything at all." Now I might have rolled my eyes at her at the time, except that my mother followed it up with another bit of wisdom; "Kill 'em with kindness. Nothing will bother them more." Okay, Mom!

I always loved my mom's subtle sense of humor, and the fact that even her little quips held important life lessons or reminders to choose happiness. Mom became known for her insights, which my friends began calling *Gladyisms.* I want to share with you a few of Glitzy Glady's most memorable *Gladyisms* — lessons that have helped me remain happy and positive throughout my life.

When you have a fight with your mate, never tell your mother or your best friend, for you'll make up, but they will forever remember what a jerk he was.

When buying a gift, give something you'd have liked to receive yourself, and you'll never go wrong.

Never hold a grudge. It's wasting valuable moments when you could be happy.

Hitch your wagon to a star and expect to go far.

When people talk to me about my life and career, I'm always surprised when they say things such as, "You seem like you have an amazingly happy life, but then, of course you would, with all the success you've had and all the amazing things you've had the chance to do." It always stops me cold when I hear that, because I don't believe that we become happy because we've become successful. I think it's the other way around. We become successful because we exude happiness and confidence. We don't become happy when we *get* to do amazing things. We *get* to do amazing things because we make those things happen. We don't become happy because we find a great mate. We attract a great mate because we are happy, fun-loving, and comfortable people.

I remember interviewing Farrah Fawcett at the height of her *Charlie's Angels* success. I asked her what she thought it was about her that had created such a media frenzy. She said, "I think it's that I have a *joie de vivre.*" Now, I will admit to you, I didn't have a clue as to what that meant at the time, but I went back to my office and looked it up. I found that it's French and it means "a love of life." Maybe it was Farrah's *joie de vivre,* her inner glow, her love of life that lit up the television screen and captivated a nation. My husband says that's crazy talk — that it was really that little red bathing suit she wore on that famous poster. But I think Farrah was on to something.

> "Success is not the key to happiness; happiness is the key to success."
> — ALBERT SCHWEITZER

Embracing that philosophy — that happiness is key to success — can change your perspective on happiness. How many people are waiting around for someone or something to come along and make them happy? You could wait forever for that!

> "Happiness resides within us, but it is up to us to unlock it."
> — UNKNOWN

People often ask what the hardest part of doing *Good Morning America* for 20 years was. I could probably cite interviews with politicians who were testy and didn't want to answer, or rock stars who were stoned and *couldn't* answer, but I think the biggest challenge was to consistently project — day

411

in and day out — a positive attitude, an energy, and exuberance for the day. I knew that my attitude was the first thing the viewer would be exposed to, even prior to the information I had to deliver.

Each morning at 7 a.m., whether I had had an argument, a disappointment, or a restless night's sleep, I needed to leave it in the dressing room and start the day with a smile. I knew how important it was to awaken the viewers with a positive outlook.

I guess I taught this lesson of positive thinking to my daughters, because my Lindsay came home one day from the sixth grade, excited over a story about the power of a positive attitude she heard from a motivational speaker who visited her school — a speaker who obviously made a big impression on her. It's become such a favorite story of mine that I often share it when giving motivational talks myself. Here's the story she told me:

A group of scientists decided to try an experiment to see if they could change a complete optimist into a pessimist, and a complete pessimist into an optimist.

They went to a preschool classroom and chose a little girl who always found the good in everything around her. When it

412

rained, she said, "Oh well, the rain is good for the flowers. It will make them grow."

Then they chose a little boy who could not find the good in anything. To him, a bright, sunny day meant that he would just be hot and sweaty. They took them both back to the laboratory and put them in two separate rooms.

The little boy's room was filled with toys, video games, trucks, cars, everything you'd imagine he could want. They left him alone for one hour and said, "Have fun."

Then they put the little girl in a room filled with nothing but horse manure, and they left her alone for an hour to see what she would do.

An hour later, they checked on the little boy, and he was just sitting there. He hadn't touched a thing.

When they asked him why he didn't play with the toys they provided, he said it was stupid. He wouldn't have time to play with everything, so he didn't play with anything.

Then they checked on the little girl.

When they walked into her room, they found her jumping around playfully in the manure and throwing it over her shoulders. When they asked her why she was doing that, she smiled and said, "With all this evidence, there's got to be a pony in here somewhere!"

Holy crap! (Pun intended.) Our attitude really can be an incredibly powerful factor in shaping how we see our world and how we are able to navigate it. Which of those children do you think you would be?

I, for one, want to be on that little girl's team!

Compared to pessimists, optimistic people are said to be more successful in school, at work, and in sports. They are more likely to be healthier, happier, more satisfied with their relationships, less likely to suffer from anxiety or depression, more resilient and in the end . . . you guessed it . . . they live longer.

According to a survey of executive recruiters at Harvard University, 85 percent of everything accomplished by Harvard students after graduation in the way of wealth, position, and status, is the result of their attitude; only 15 percent is the result of their aptitude or ability. I definitely think my positive attitude and my belief in my abilities, as well as in my future, have played a key role in helping me get to the top of my field.

> "Act as if you are already happy, and that will tend to make you happy."
> — DALE CARNEGIE

The Power of Positive

Let's face it — it isn't always easy to keep our focus on the positive in today's complex world. But the effort is so worth it! It challenges us to reframe the way we look at any given situation.

Let's say we're sitting in our car in terrible traffic. There are vehicles ahead and behind us for as far as we can see. Ugh! Reacting negatively and getting upset is not going to make the guy in front of us move any faster. Not even if you flip him the bird.

I've always thought that someone should come up with a small device for our cars that would sit on our dashboard where it would be completely visible to other drivers. It would light up and display messages, ranging from "I'm not a mind-reader — where's your turn signal?!" and "Honk if you like my parking," (especially funny when you're sitting still on the freeway) to "Hey, there's a lane for that!" (Something direct and generic enough for speedsters, road hogs, and even nosepickers!)

But until the day that device gets made and sold, we should make the most of our time in annoying traffic jams amusing ourselves in more constructive ways, such as listening to our favorite playlist or the next chapter of an audiobook. It can actually make us feel like we've slipped in a little of that *me time* we've been craving. What a difference that could make in our day!

> "Life is a mirror; if you frown
> at it, it frowns back;
> if you smile, it returns the greeting."
> — WILLIAM THACKERAY

The Power of a Smile!

Did you know that the best prescription for beating the blues could be as simple as smiling or laughing? I'm not kidding. According to researchers at Clark University in Worcester, Massachusetts, sometimes we should just force ourselves to grin and bear it, literally. The students in their study were told to assume happy, sad, or angry facial expressions and postures for four minutes.

The researchers found that participating students maintained those moods for up to one hour later. James Laird, Ph.D., Clark University Professor of Psychology and coauthor of the study, said they are not exactly sure why it happens but one theory is that acting happy forces our brain to evoke good memories, which in turn puts us in a better mood. Then we smile, and people smile back — it's a crazy good chain reaction. You might say it increases our face value. Scowling, on the other hand, makes us feel angrier, by conjuring up bad memories. That sourpuss face can then affect how others see us or even how they perceive we feel about them. You can see where this is going.

> "People who keep stiff upper lips,
> find that it's damn hard to smile."
> — JUDITH GUEST

The Power of Laughter

Something as simple as laughing can reduce anxiety, lower our blood pressure, and give us more energy. The effects of just two minutes of hearty laughter have been likened to the effects of 10 minutes on a rowing machine. So doesn't that make laughter an aerobic activity?! Now, that's exercise that everyone should be able to get behind!

> "Laughter is the brush that sweeps away
> the cobwebs of the heart."
> — MORT WALKER

There is actually such a thing as humor

therapy, and it is part of a growing field of medicine called psychoneuroimmunology. This is the study of the relationship between the emotional and the physical. While we've known for ages that stress weakens the body's overall condition, we are now learning that the opposite is also true: feel-good emotions have a positive impact on our health. I know a comedian who tells me she can go to a club exhausted and down in the dumps, but once she's on stage telling jokes and creating laughter, she instantly becomes energized and is actually happy herself.

It's been said that laughter is potent enough to ward off colds, stifle the flu, and help us sleep better. That's right, good old-fashioned laughter is getting a lot of attention these days for its role in boosting the immune system. According to a study from Indiana State University, laughter can boost the immune system by up to 40 percent. It has to do with the diaphragmatic breathing that happens when we laugh hard. It causes lymphatic fluid to move 10 to 15 times harder and faster than it does ordinarily. The increased flow elevates the number of lymphocytes circulating in the blood, which, in turn, creates better immunity toward disease. In fact, it has also been found that laughter can increase the production of our

418

bodies' killer cells that attack some forms of cancer.

Researchers say we can't be physically tense if we are laughing. A good laugh provides a cathartic release, a cleansing of emotions, and a release of emotional tension. Even after the laughter has ended, body tensions continue to decrease. All this gives new meaning to the phrase "fall down laughing," as smiling and laughing seem to be the ultimate relaxation and stress management technique. So the next time you're feeling sad or stressed, flash a big smile or give a hearty laugh and feel the tension melt away.

> "A person without humor is like a car without shock absorbers."
> — UNKNOWN

The Power of Rejuvenation
Life is all about balance. You don't always need to be getting stuff done. Sometimes it's perfectly okay, and absolutely necessary, to shut down, kick back, and do nothing. Remember what always helped when our kids got all wound up and whacked out? We gave them a *time-out.* A period of time to back it down and to calmly reflect. Well, I'm going to suggest that we give ourselves

419

the same kind of "time-out" to . . . wait for it . . . step back, calm down, and reflect. I had a tough time coming to grips with this concept at first. I've always had a tendency to speed through life at 100 mph and felt guilty whenever I kicked back. It took some doing to wake up to the benefits of powering down, but I finally have. What I've learned is that "me time" isn't a dirty word at all.

Studies have shown that monks tend to live longer than most people because with practiced meditation they are able to slow down their heart rate and thus the aging process. We can all take a lesson from them and carve out some time each day to try meditation, either on our own or with the guidance of an app, to help us to slow our breathing, heart rate, and to keep the day's stresses out of focus. Yoga and Pilates are also recommended for reducing stress (I'm dying to take up both), as is something as simple as listening to music — not necessarily the music your teenaged kids might be listening to — but soothing sounds have been found to have an influence on our emotions as well as our brains.

So hit pause, stretch out, relax, breathe, and meditate. All have been shown to extend our healthy years and add quality to our lives. Sometimes the best prescription for good health is a little rest and play. I actually look forward to my time-outs now.

The Power of No

This has always been a tough one for me. As I've said before, I'm a pleaser. I know it. I'm not alone on this though, I think women are naturally wired to say "Yes" and then we pride ourselves in being there for everyone in our lives. However, learning to say "No" and stop biting off more than we can chew goes a long way in finding our own happiness. Learning to say "No" is almost like building up a muscle. At first, when we say it, we tend to feel bad (maybe even sore about it), but the more we do it and get used to it, the better we feel!

Let's all remember this: "No" is a complete sentence!

The Power of Adventure

I love to travel, and I love the fact that travel is actually good for us!! I recently interviewed John Tierney, *New York Times* science columnist, about how travel impacts our health and wellness. Tierney told me, "If we want to be happier, we're better off spending our money on new experiences instead of new stuff at the store." I loved that piece of advice.

According to Tierney, who writes about science and lifestyles in terms of their scientific impact on a person's well-being, people who take more vacations tend to be healthier both physically and mentally. They have fewer heart attacks, suffer less from depression, and they're more productive when they go back to work.

Travel forces us to exercise our mental muscles. We've got to make plans, make decisions, and absorb a ton of new information both before and during the trip. We're solving a series of puzzles and researchers tell us that these real-world puzzles are a better mental workout than a daily crossword puzzle, because they're unfamiliar and more challenging, keep our mental circuits healthy, and they build new connections in the brain.

> "My favorite thing is to go where I've never been."
> — DIANE ARBUS

Travel also helps us embrace new cultures and new foods, which stimulates the brain's dopamine system — the same system that gets stimulated when we fall in love. I knew there was a reason why I adore travel so

422

much! So never let an adventure pass you by and if people tease you for constantly being on the go, tell them it's doctor's orders. It's a great Rx for more energy, optimism, and happiness! I haven't been everywhere, but it's on my bucket list.

> "Adventure is worthwhile in itself."
> — AMELIA EARHART

The Power of Connection

One of the fundamental human drivers is what psychologists call *the need to belong.* We're social animals drawn to being part of a group. It's why, when we explore our family roots, our life can feel so much more meaningful. We see ourselves as part of this much larger group that goes way back in time.

I've found that as I have grown older, I have become more interested in my family history. Psychologists used to think that nostalgia was a sign of depression, suggesting that you're living in the past to avoid the present. but they've now come to see exploring one's family connections as one of the surest ways to boost a person's happiness.

Like millions of others, one of my guilty pleasures is spending hours on

Ancestry.com. More and more people are exploring their ancestry these days and travelling with the express purpose of connecting with their family origins. It's one of the fastest growing trends in travel. I remember when *Good Morning America* broadcast live from Australia, the researchers on our production helped me search for some of my dad's relatives since he had been born in Sydney. We found a few of them and brought them on the show. It was a bit odd to meet strangers to whom I was so directly related, but I learned so much about my dad's side of the family that I'd been totally unaware of since we lived so far from one another.

Again, when GMA broadcast live from Kilkenny, Ireland, the researchers learned of a nearby castle that was in my family. It's called Castle Blunden.

I guess now I need to explain that I was born Joan *Blunden.*

When I moved to New York City in my mid-20s to work at WABC TV as a reporter, the news director told me that I needed to change my name. He said that New York TV critics were ruthless and could have a heyday playing around with my name and referring to me as a Blunder. I couldn't argue with him since I clearly remembered going out to dinner with my family as a child, and my dad leaving his name with the hostess only to hear them call out when our table was ready "Dr. Blunder, party of four." It used to irritate my dad to no end; after all, he was a surgeon, and they don't make blunders! It was decided that I'd simply drop the B and become Joan Lunden. Calling my mom that night to tell her, just as my career on TV was beginning to take off, that I was changing my name was not one of the easiest calls I've ever made.

So again, GMA researchers had found family members on my dad's side, but this time they lived in a castle! I couldn't wait to see it. Sir William Blunden and his wife Lady Pamela Blunden had taken over the place and raised six daughters there. Yes, I did just say "Sir William Blunden." No, that doesn't make me a lady or a princess by lineage. Darn. But I was able to learn that in the late 1700s there were two Blunden brothers who lived in England. Both were made Lords by the King of England. One set off for Australia (that's the brother from whom I descend) and the other, Sir John Blunden, went to Ireland. The castle was originally a 13-bedroom, 2-bathroom house. (I hope they all had strong bladders. LOL.) When I visited the castle in 1991, Sir William had already passed away, but I got to spend some time with Lady Pamela who gave me the inside story on having six daughters when you really need a son to inherit the title and the castle. She told me that after having four girls, the couple decided to give it one more try for a male heir, and voila they had twin girls! Can you imagine? As titles descended only through male lines at that time, the title — and eventually the castle — passed to William's brother, and then to nephew Patrick who now lives there and has been renovating the castle for the past 10 years. It is currently a 9-bedroom, 9-bathroom home. (That sounds more like it.)

But don't lust over the idea of living in a castle. It not only lacked most modern innovations (such as central heat and air conditioning), it cost a fortune to operate and had created a financial struggle for its occupants for decades. However, I found out a lot about my ancestors while there and Lady Pamela invited our GMA cameras to tour the castle, which made for a great story!

If you're interested in finding out more about your family provenance, the way I started was by talking to relatives and then going online to discover more about the specific towns or areas where our ancestors had settled. In the end, I learned so much about the complicated early history of England and Ireland, first from my new-found kin and then by reading about the local history and culture back at the time my family migrated from England to the Kilkenny area. It's been so much fun, and best of all, it's provided me with that sense of belonging that is so essential to our inner peace.

"You don't stop laughing when
you grow old,
you grow old when you stop laughing."
— GEORGE BERNARD SHAW

CHAPTER 26
I WANT TO BE CREMATED; IT'S MY LAST CHANCE FOR A SMOKIN' HOT BODY

"When I asked for a smoking hot body menopause was not what I had in mind."

— UNKNOWN

I want to go on record right now: When I pass, I'd like to go out in my favorite little black dress, or as my daughters say, my LBD, and I want my stylist, Emir, to do my hair and my makeup for my last act. I want my eulogy to be filled with some good knee-slapping humor. I'm serious! I don't want people crying; it makes our mascara run.

All joking aside though, I'm enough of a control freak that I would like to be able to exercise some power over how I'll look and what will be said about me at my funeral. You know, we can have that kind of power if we take control and make our requests known.

This is where I'm going to suggest that we write *our own* obituary and eulogy.

Wait! Don't close the book!

Hear me out . . .

I know it sounds a little strange, but stick with me, because I've found that these exercises can have a profound effect on us. They require us to step back and take stock of our life. All of it — our loves, our work, our passions, and our accomplishments. But it's not just about the successes in our life; it's also about how we've treated people along the way. It is a retrospective of our existence that allows us to review our legacy thus far and determine how we want to proceed in the years going forward.

If we want to be remembered as compassionate and always there for others, we have today and every day hereafter to make that happen. If we want to be remembered as an advocate for people or a worthy cause, then all we have to do is get busy in that regard now. Or if you simply want to be remembered as a lighthearted, happy-go-lucky person who made people smile and was always the life of the party, then by all means, pursue that delightful path. Let your joyful light lead the way.

We can all use a little guidance in our lives and sometimes it's better to look inward for that enlightenment than it is to look outward. I believe that this kind of reflective exercise can give us a new kind of power over both our day-to-day lives and our legacy.

Quite honestly, I did not come up with this idea myself. I first heard about it at an event at the Superdome in New Orleans where I was booked to speak at a huge motivational conference. While I was waiting for my turn in the program, I stood backstage watching one of the other speakers, inspirational author Stephen Covey, who wrote *The Seven Habits of Highly Effective People.* I had never heard him speak before this occasion, but he had me and the audience of over 25,000 people completely captivated. He asked everyone to close their eyes and imagine themselves at a funeral . . . their own funeral.

"Can you picture it?" he asked. "Are you there?" I swear to God, this guy Covey was good. I was totally there, and I assume all the other people in the arena who had their eyes closed were too. From that point on, he led one of the most remarkable guided sessions I'd ever heard.

Through a series of really penetrating questions, as only he can ask them, Covey directed us all to envision people walking by us as we lay motionless in our own casket. I was so transported that I actually saw myself tucked into a white coffin lined in matching soft, white satin — not that I'm requesting a white casket when my time comes. Well, maybe.

You could have heard a pin drop in that enormous stadium. Covey spoke slowly, reverently, the way you'd imagine a psychiatrist speaking to you. His carefully phrased narrative stoked our inner thoughts and escorted us deeper into the images our mind conjured. We were all mesmerized as he took us through the exercise of imagining what the people in our lives were saying about us

"One by one, people are filing by," said Covey. "Hey, look who's coming now." He slowly paraded people from different parts of our life past us: friends, neighbors, and co-workers. "Do you think they're fondly remembering your kindness and dedication to others or do you think they're worried about where you might be heading now?" asked Covey. He let a minute or two pass before speaking each time, almost forcing us to fill the empty space with truthful answers to his questions. Then it was time for our family members to pass by our casket. The questions he asked about what they would be thinking and feeling stopped me in my tracks.

It was the most sobering visualization exercise I'd ever experienced. I would go so far as to say it was powerfully transformative. It was a wake-up call, and God only knows, you wanted to wake up from this exercise.

> "What you are, is God's gift to you.
> What you do with that, is your gift to God."
> — HANS URS VON BALTHASAR

Write the Ending to Your Own Story

Just in case creative writing wasn't your favorite class in school, I did a little research and found some incredibly helpful advice to make this next part of the assignment — the obit-writing part — a little less daunting. Since an obituary is a concise, concentrated review of one's life, I discovered that it's easier to get started if you look at your Facebook page. (I'm assuming that most of us have one of those.)

It's actually a brilliant concept, as so many of us have become self-published documenters of our lives on our various social media platforms. In fact, this exercise will likely be smoother if you approach it as you would approach any social media posting.

Just look at what you've already written in

the "about me" section. You should find the following categories:

Work and education
Places you've lived
Contact and basic info
Family and relationships
Details about you
Life events

Cut and paste how you've already presented yourself onto a blank document and now you've got the basics down. If you are anything like me, you probably write about your life, your family, your pursuits, and your adventures with relative openness on your social media platforms. To bolster what you have in your obit so far, peruse your timeline and add whatever jumps out at you as really representing *you*. There you have it — a brief and concentrated review of your life. Don't think of it so much as your obit, but rather as your final selfie!

Now it's time to turn your attention to your eulogy, which is a much more comprehensive account of who you are and how you have lived your life. Okay, some of you may be a bit back on your heels about attempting this final stage of the exercise, but at the very least, I suggest that you collect the information about yourself that you would like included in your eulogy, and give it to whomever will be left with the task of actually writing the final version and delivering it.

Think of your eulogy as the story of your life. It's not a job resume. It's a colorful portrait of who you are as a person. Remember how I described my mom as having an effervescent personality, how when she left a room you felt her presence, kind of like a shooting star leaves a trail. Try to include descriptive phrases like that and don't be afraid to be humorous. Those attending your funeral will greatly appreciate some light moments. This is your chance to talk about your life dreams, your achievements, and the challenges you've overcome.

Incidentally, if you are reading this right now and saying to yourself under your breath, "Oh, there's really nothing important to say about my life," I want you to stop that right now. *Everyone has a story worth telling.*

Frankly, that is exactly what this exercise is all about. It allows us to feel satisfaction and appreciation for what we've done in our lives, while also providing an opportunity to recognize what we still want to do before our eulogy is ever read aloud.

434

Some of you probably have some reservations about considering your own mortality, but I think this exercise is an interesting and a safe way to approach our passing in terms of the life we've lived. Of course, many people regularly journal and find it quite useful in tracking their life experiences and the various successes, challenges and decisions that have brought meaning to their lives.

This kind of life review is a unique chance to applaud our accomplishments, even if perhaps they weren't exactly what we set out to do. I always thought I'd be a doctor like my dad was and have occasionally questioned if I should have worked harder to accomplish that goal. Not living up to that expectation has led to moments of disappointment.

Going through this exercise allowed me to revel in what I *have* accomplished in the area of health advocacy. I now recognize that there are many ways to help others live healthy, productive, and long lives. A friend once told me that no one is actually dead until the ripples they created in the world die away. I'd like to think that the ripples my father made during his time on earth are still very much alive and active in me today.

"I may not have gone where I intended to go, but I think I have ended up where I NEEDED to be."
— DOUGLAS ADAMS
AUTHOR OF *THE LONG DARK TEA-TIME OF THE SOUL*

So stop and think about your life. Were you a loving wife? A devoted mother? A supportive friend? Or perhaps you were someone's devoted child. The personal story you write will be a precious gift for your loved ones. In fact, it may even help them get to know and understand you better. Your story can be read by your children, and their children, and on down through the generations long after you're gone.

Don't get me wrong — I am not focusing on this because I am a pessimistic, morose, doomsday kind of person. I am not fixated on my death or the probability of my cancer coming back. I consider myself cured of cancer, and I am not expecting it to return at all.

Actually, the idea of writing an obituary for myself has been less about dying and more about living. It's all been about how I'm using my time on this earth. This made me think about hearing my dad's eulogy.

When My Dad Died

My first experience with obituary writing came at a very young age. As I mentioned earlier, I was 13 when my dad was tragically killed in an airplane crash. My mom had to write his obituary. I remember her sitting down with one of those long yellow legal pads, tears streaming down her face as she began committing her memories to paper.

By the end, my mom had wiped her eyes, pulled herself together, gathered renewed strength, and told my brother and me that we should find comfort in how admired and respected our father was and by the incredible outpouring of love we were witnessing. So many people attended the funeral that the church had to pipe the sound outside to the crowd of mourners who couldn't get inside the church.

Writing about my father's life and accomplishments and what he had meant to friends, family, colleagues, and to everyone in our community turned out to be incredibly therapeutic for my mom.

Only a week before his passing, we had celebrated my mom's and my brother's birthdays (January 15 and 20, respectively). My dad had flown to Los Angeles to speak at a cancer convention in a brand-new plane he'd just purchased. On January 17, he was to fly home to join us for the celebratory weekend. When he called my mom from LA, he said that he loved the new plane but had experienced some trouble with the radio and had the electronics worked on at the airport while he was at the convention.

The weather was stormy, so Dad filed a VFR (Visual Flight Rules) flight plan at the airport. Thirty minutes after takeoff, air traffic controllers lost contact with the plane. It was after midnight when a police officer came to the door to tell Mom that Dad's plane was thought to have gone down in Malibu Canyon. Officials would begin the search in the morning.

The next day friends began arriving to console my mother, and then the dreaded news came. Search planes had found the wreckage against a mountainside. I remember seeing an article in the newspaper about my dad's death with a fuzzy black-and-white photo of the crash site on California's Malibu mountainside. As much as I didn't want to think about it, I still wanted to understand more about what happened. Frankly, I couldn't help but wonder how much of the plane was left after it hit the mountain. And what about my dad? I didn't want to ask my mom; she was so upset.

One day before the funeral, I overheard

her asking if she would be able to look at Dad inside the casket and a friend told her that it wasn't possible because the impact of the crash was too severe. The mind works in crazy ways. I thought to myself, *If there was no body to see, then maybe he walked away after the crash, had amnesia, and couldn't find his way back to us.* That thought, as terrible as it was, gave me hope that someday he would remember who he was and would come home.

It took years for me to let go of that thinking. I've always wondered about it. Then last year I received the following message on Facebook:

"Joan, with a lump in my throat I heard you speak of your father's death. My husband was one of the deputies with the LA County Sheriff's Department who retrieved your father's body from the wreckage. My husband came home that night extremely upset. Please know we never forgot about that awful accident, and only recently when I heard you speak on a program, did I realize the connection. I'm thinking of you. God bless you."

Reading that woman's message took me back to that day when we heard that the wreckage of the plane had been found and that my dad was dead. It took me back to that scene in my living room, sitting with my brother while my mom read us the obituary she'd written, asking us for any suggestions. I don't remember adding anything, but I do remember being in awe of all of my father's accomplishments that my mother read them aloud.

I think it became indelibly imprinted somewhere in my brain that my goal in life should be to have someone write an obituary like that about me someday. Surely that's what ignited my burning desire to become a doctor or to do something in my life that would have made an impact in the world.

Years later, my mom would write another obituary — her own.

I'm serious. My mom sat down, again with a pen and a long yellow legal pad, and said, "I want to write my obituary because I know what I am proud of in my life and I want to be in charge of what will be said at my Bon Voyage party." You had to love the way my mom looked at life, and even at her passing. By the way, she did not do this when she was in her 90s or even her 80s. No, she was barely 70 at the time but said, "You never know when your time is going to come, and I want this obituary and eulogy in your files."

Together, we — well, mainly Mom — proceeded to write her life story the way she wanted it to be remembered. She actually went a bit further than that; she produced the entire funeral as a grand event! She provided a guest list and told me what she would like to wear, in the casket, that is. She wanted to be seen in her nicest ivory St. John knit pant suit with gold trim and a gold cami, and her favorite gold shoes.

Mom absolutely wanted her long-time hairdresser, Jo Avilla, to do her hair and makeup for the event. Yes, I did just say *the event,* because that's what she called it. She also requested that a certain friend with a beautiful voice sing that day and she even gave me her song choices. Most importantly, she wanted it to be an upbeat celebration. She did *not* want it to be sad or morose. It was quite a production she had put together — almost primetime worthy.

When My Mom Died, We Celebrated Her Life

When my mom passed away at almost 95, I went through my files and found that eulogy that she'd written along with her *show rundown.* I'm serious, it was really like a *show*

441

rundown! I couldn't contact the woman she'd hoped would sing at her farewell event because she'd passed away, but I was able to manage everything else my mom had requested for this occasion.

You can bet that she was wearing her ivory St. John knit pant suit with the gold trim and those gold shoes of hers while she was nestled into her gold casket. Oh yes, I did. I bought her a gold casket. Come on, how could I not? I even included her cherished gold Chanel handbag, the one that she had purchased on sale during one of her many trips to New York City. The one she proudly carried *everywhere* with her.

When I returned to New York after the funeral and told a group of my friends about my mom's Bon Voyage party and how I made sure to bury her with all of her favorite things, one of my friends asked incredulously, "Wait, did you just say that you put a gold Chanel handbag into the casket? Are you kidding? You didn't keep it?" Catching herself, she added, "I mean, of course, to remember your mother by."

Hey, I put that Chanel purse in mom's casket because you never know; she may have use for it up there. If anyone were to throw a party upon arrival in heaven, it would be her, and she'll want to be dressed to the nines when meeting her maker!

I will tell you that in a time of sadness when a loved one passes, it is difficult to attend to such details. The fact that my mom had already told me what she wanted said in her obituary and in her eulogy was so helpful and comforting.

I didn't read the eulogy my mom had written word for word, since I had a few loving things to add. I'd like to share with you what I read to those attending the funeral of my inimitable mom, Glitzy Glady.

EULOGY FOR GLADY B

We are here today to celebrate the life of Glady Blunden, also known as Glitzy Glady. Mom was my own personal Guru of positive thinking and living out your dreams. In fact, a lot of my friends thought Gandhi may have raised me because I'm always pulling another "Gladyism" out of my hat, like:

The word "impossible" isn't in our dictionary.

Can't is a four-letter word.

Have at least one big party every year so you really clean your house.

443

(and my personal favorite)

Tan fat is better than white fat.

Glady always saw the glass half-full and her positive outlook was contagious. Glitzy Glady would want that joyful happy spirit that she always emanated to be alive and well here today, for she lived a full and wonderful life, not void of adversity or sadness, but bounding with energy and enthusiasm.

Mom was born on a farm in North Dakota, and when she and her siblings weren't at school in their one-room schoolhouse, they were doing their farm chores. Mom would come to the dinner table at night, all dolled up in a dress with a dainty white hanky in hand. Her father, who was a gruff farmer, would look at her puzzled and ask, "Who you trying to kid 'farm' girl? Who do you think you're going to impress?" Mom would look at him and say, "Me. I'm trying to impress upon myself that my life can be better than this." Mom never did mince words.

Mom had big dreams for her life, even as a young girl. At 16, Glady began working as a waitress earning $1 a day plus tips, so she learned quickly the importance of making a good first impression. She worked 2 shifts a day and went to business school to learn to operate a Comptometer — an accounting machine that was later replaced by the adding machine, which was, of course, later replaced by the computer.

She used her new skill to get a job at Shell Oil Company and made lots of friends with her new co-workers. One new friend invited mom to join her and her date for dinner. That girl made a really big mistake! Her date was a handsome doctor and her friend had been pushing him hard to get married. Glady, on the other hand, was wide-eyed and excited about building a career, which was intriguing to young Dr. Erle Blunden. And yes, it wasn't long before they were dating steadily.

Glady, too, was quite intrigued with this young doctor who was also an avid private pilot and would fly her around in his own airplane. The two quickly became serious, but Erle announced that he would only marry her if she too took flying lessons and got her pilot's license. He wanted assurance that she would become his co-pilot for life. Needless to say, Mom took his challenge!

In February of 1948, they flew off to Las Vegas to get married, with Glady as his licensed co-pilot. Mom wanted to start a family but miscarried several times — so they decided to adopt. I'd like to tell you this part of the story, in my mom's own words.

"A colleague of Erle's called to say that he had just delivered a baby who was up for adoption, a stunning little boy. We went to the hospital nursery to look at the baby boy who was smiling and seemed to just be waiting for us.

"So with baby wrapped in a blanket, we headed for home stopping at a pharmacy to get the necessary baby feeding supplies. I carried him around Fair Oaks to see all of our friends but soon I found I wasn't feeling well — my lady friends came to the house to make me a baby shower — but I stayed in bed. Did I have the flu? I was so nauseated! What a surprise when we discovered that I was actually pregnant. On September 19, 1950, I delivered a little girl. Just 7 months

and 29 days apart — I wanted to name them like twins, Jeffrey Erle and Joanie Elise, same initials. My world was now complete."

Mom worked hard to make sure that we were exposed to a lot — theater, ballet, trips around the U.S. and to foreign countries. She wanted us to see the world, to "broaden our horizons" — those were *her* words.

Mom constantly told me that I would do great things with my life. Those were positive affirmations that had a long-term effect. I once heard that children are likely to live up to what you believe of them. I have always felt that I am strong because a strong woman raised me.

I remember being a teenager and dissing my mom and, yes, rolling my eyes. I also remember that when she would be at her wits' end with me, an hour later she would come into my room and in her most cheerful voice she would offer up some invitation that was just too darn good to pass up. In my case, it probably involved shopping. My mom's goal was to provide a teaching moment for me; she wanted me

447

to realize that the troubling moment had passed and was forgotten. She wanted me to see that she had let go of it and we were going to move on. Thank you, Mom, for that priceless lesson.

My mom was living a charmed life until January of 1964, when Dad's plane went down in Malibu Canyon. Mom was left with two young teenagers to raise. Watching my mom take over as a single parent when my dad died, taught me how to be strong and resilient in life. My dad had handled all the business in our family, and my mom had raised us. But she had to figure out how to carry on in order to take care of us kids. Mom had to quickly become a sharp businessperson. She got her Realtor's license and began selling residential real estate.

Mom managed to raise Jeff and me and keep our lives essentially the same as if my dad wasn't gone. We stayed in our house and we also continued to travel. I feel fortunate to have had a parent who exposed us to the world, who believed that we could succeed, and who told us again and again that we could achieve great things.

When we see our mom exhibit strength, it makes us strong. When we see our mom let things roll off her back, it teaches us patience and compassion. When we see our mom challenge herself and dare to try new things, it teaches us that we, too, can expect greater things of ourselves. It teaches us not to create limits, but to believe that we can accomplish more than even we might think.

My mom also continually talked about my dad, and how he had saved so many lives and taken care of so many families. That, too, influenced our expectations of what we should do with our lives.

Mom had a tremendous impact on my life — on my career and success. So it has been my pleasure in the past few decades to try to make her life the best that I could make it — well, maybe a few less Rolexes and world cruises. But Glady lived life to the fullest. She savored every moment, she did it all, she had no regrets, and she was so very appreciative of it all.

I want you to know that I made sure that today Glady B still looked "all gussied up," as she would say. She is wearing the gold and white outfit just as she requested for this occasion along with gold shoes and her gold Chanel bag.

I will confess that when I took her "going away outfit" as she called it, to the funeral director, I had one little problem. These past few years have been what some might call the "Depends years" so I couldn't find any of her underwear. One of her nice caregivers quickly ran to her room to get a pair that she had just purchased. That was so nice; however, I felt I needed to explain as I handed the bikini under-pants to the funeral director with her outfit. I told him, when my mom goes through the Pearly gates and meets back up with Dr. Blunden and he sees those bikini briefs, she's going to have some explain-ing to do. Of course, she's going to say, "Swear to God, I don't know where these came from."

Heaven will never be the same now that Glitzy Glady's there.

CHAPTER 27
IT'S NEVER TOO LATE TO BE THE PERSON YOU WANT TO BE

"We are each gifted in a unique and important way. It is our privilege and our adventure to discover our own special light."

— MARY DUNBAR

The first time I really faced my mortality was when I was diagnosed with breast cancer. As I contemplated the real possibility of not beating the cancer and what would transpire in the days and years after I was gone, my mind was flooded with concerning thoughts. I worried about my husband and how he would have to handle our hectic life raising our children alone, and of course, I worried about all of my kids — the young ones and the fully grown ones, and how they wouldn't have me around for important events in their lives.

Facing my own mortality also made me ponder the imprint I was leaving on the

451

world. If I was to get more years or maybe even more decades if all went well, what should I get busy doing to make a difference?

It's Never Too Late to Take Control of Your Legacy

It's never too late to start building the lasting reputation for which you'd like to be remembered. It's never too late for us to begin changing our ways and our behaviors, so that we influence the words that will be used to describe us in our eulogy.

> "Life isn't about finding yourself. It's about creating yourself."
> — GEORGE BERNARD SHAW

I remember listening to the eulogy at the funeral for my husband's grandmother Rosie. She had been a colorful character, a real matriarch of her family, and was being fondly remembered.

The person giving Nana Rosie's eulogy read a poem called "The Dash" by Linda Ellis. It's a favorite of mine. It asks how the person has lived their life between their birth and their passing, which is represented by that dash on our tombstone. I'd heard it before, but this time I seemed to be hearing the words in a more profound way, especially the following two lines.

"So think about this long and hard.
Are there things you'd like to change?
For you never know how much time is
left, that can still be rearranged."

I found those words to be intensely powerful. The essence of "The Dash" can serve to guide our behavior by helping us to imagine what people will say about us as they remember us at our funeral and what they will be thinking as they walk by our coffin for one last goodbye.

I'm not trying to be morbid, but I am trying to be blunt.

This stage of life allows us to adjourn briefly and look back with a bit of wonder at what has passed and what is yet to come. To take a true and accurate measurement of our contributions large and small. This discovery — this permission to reflect and take pride in a life well-lived — is the silver lining of aging.

So how about you?

What can you learn about yourself, your dreams, and your hopes for your future by engaging in this kind of contemplation?

What would you like written on your

tombstone?

As for my tombstone, I'd be happy if it simply read:

> She was classy, sassy, and a bit
> bad-assy.

ACKNOWLEDGMENTS

For six years this book has had a hold on me. I knew it needed to be written but something always seemed to get in the way. It changed in name, and even in content and direction, but once I settled into aging as its theme, the chapters simply fell out of my head and onto the page.

It is Laura Morton whom I really have to thank for the book as you see it. Laura has been my co-author on several books — in fact, we started this writing thing together with our first book, *Healthy Cooking with Joan Lunden* in 1996, then *Healthy Living with Joan Lunden,* and then again a few years ago to write *Had I Known*. When I spoke to Laura about working with me on this book, she told me that her commitment to other projects didn't leave her the time to say yes. I was disappointed because I've always had a sense of comfort working with Laura, knowing that in the end, we'd end up with a terrific book. What Laura was secretly doing was challenging me to write the entire book myself. She knew I had the capability and slowly pushed me into it. Thank you for that, Laura. I had so much fun writing this one. I didn't hold back; in fact, with your encouragement, I gave myself permission to be funny, which made the whole experience even better.

She joked that she'd written a book about breast cancer with me and then ended up getting breast cancer, so she wasn't sure how she felt about writing a book on aging! Once Laura saw that I had risen to her challenge and completed the book, she came on board to do her magic.

She introduced me to a wonderful publisher, Jonathan Merkh, founder of Forefront Books, who fell in love with the book right away and who has been a cheerleader and mentor to me throughout this process. Jonathan, I've loved working with you, and I look forward to doing many more books together.

And thank you to our partner, Simon & Schuster. I appreciate all the work that everyone at S&S has done bringing everything together, printing, distributing, and supporting this book.

Once the writing was completed on the

book, we turned the manuscript over to the very capable hands of Hope Innelli, our line editor. Hope, thank you for your diligence, understanding of my voice, and your commitment to excellence. You came very highly recommended and did not disappoint. We also brought on one of the funniest women we could find, comedienne Lynne Koplitz. Whereas Hope was kind of like having an angel on one of my shoulders, checking to keep my humor in line, Lynn was on the other shoulder, egging me on. Together, we struck the perfect balance . . . I think.

I want to thank our team at Forefront books, especially Bruce Gore, for your wonderful cover design and Bill Kersey, for the beautiful interior design. Thank you, Billie Brownell, for your wonderful copyediting and production assistance.

Writing has often been called a lonely process; however, I've had wonderful assistance researching and writing this book from a terrific group of women who work with me at Joan Lunden Productions. They've helped me track down answers and truths so that we could pass them on to my readership. At the helm has been Lindsay Weinberg, my VP in charge of my office and career. I'd call Lindsay my right hand — but she's also been like my left brain for the past 10 years. But wait, there's more; Lindsay also happens to be one of my daughters and one of my best friends. It's an amazing gift in life when one of your children joins you in your life passion. Thank you so much, Lindsay, for your hard work, your loyalty, for always protecting me . . . and for telling me when my skirt is too short . . . for my age. And to the other ladies in my production office, Nicole Scaramuzzo, Elaine Capillo and Ali Knopf, thank you for all your research efforts and for humoring me each time I said, "Can we all give the manuscript just one more read?"

I also want to acknowledge all the women who took part in my focus group where we discussed anything and everything that an aging woman might experience. It was a no-holds-barred conversation that made us laugh and cry. It helped me better understand which changes in our body and brain concerned you the most and what you felt you'd like to learn. Your presence and your comments helped me to stay on point and answer the questions that most concerned you. And, of course, I got a couple great one-liners from you.

For all the health professionals who made themselves available to answer my endless questions, I give you my deepest appreciation. I know how busy you are, and I applaud your determination to reach out and help me so that you could help empower women with the knowledge that they need.

When it was time to design the cover of the book, we found a talented photographer, Robbie Quinn, to shoot the image. I wanted to include a lot of humor in this book, and I knew that a quirky cover would reflect that. We told Robbie that our intention was to get away from the usual "glamour shot" that people were used to seeing of me; we were looking for a shot that was unlike anything I'd done before. It needed to match the personality within the pages. Robbie brought his own perspective to the job, which helped him capture an image that made us all smile.

Of course, it can only be a good photograph if you have a good make-up artist and hairstylist. I have that in Emir Pehilj, make-up artist and hairstylist extraordinaire. Emir is always there to make sure I'm camera ready. Emir is such an amazing talent and is also a dear friend, it is a treat to have him on the road with me. And to Bruce Gore, our wonderful art director, who put it all together to produce the final cover, I thank you.

When the project was ready to introduce

to the world, my longtime friend and colleague Elise Silvestri managed the press strategy. Elise and I have worked together for more decades than we will likely admit; she was my very first assistant when I began at *Good Morning America* in 1980. She has also worked with me on other books and continues to be a touchstone in my life.

A very special thanks to my family, who were so understanding about my passion for this project. Well, Max, Kate, Kim, and Jack were understanding as long as I still made myself available to help with writing and editing school essays. My older daughters Jamie, Lindsay, and Sarah are my cheerleaders but also my voices of reason who will tell me, "Mom, you can't say that."

And finally, the love of my life, my husband, Jeff, is without fail always supportive of my endeavors and has been incredibly patient with the writing process. Sorry, sweetheart, for all the nights I stayed up until the wee hours with my late-night writing. I love you.

INDEX

absentmindedness. *See* memory loss
adrenaline, 100–101, 236–37, 242, 244,
    251, 304
advantages of still having parents, 65–72
aerobic activity, 97, 192–94, 198, 241, 375,
    417
age, defined, 23–36, 44–45, 48–59
age, measuring, 26–42, 366
ageism, 15–16
age spots, 41
aging, attitudes on, 14–15, 16, 29, 44–45,
    77–87, 360–77
aging, signs of, 37–47
alcohol, 95, 105, 131, 147, 235–36, 237,
    243, 262–63, 268, 276
Alzheimer's, 94, 103, 104, 106, 176,
    193–94
amyloid, 104
andropause, 131–32
antioxidants, 103, 222, 224, 268, 303

sex, 134–40, 264. *See also* vaginal
    discomfort
shame, 16
signs of aging, 37–47
skin care, 41–42, 218, 221, 248
skin exam, 162–63
sleep, 104, 217–18, 227, 235, 246–65, 268,
    297, 301, 303–305, 322, 386, 418
sleep disorders, 129, 139, 150, 247–248,
    250–51, 267
smiling, 416–17. *See also* laughter
smoking, 73–74, 94–95, 105, 123, 131,
    147, 148–49, 190, 243, 262–63, 268,
    276, 382
social connection, 101–103, 374, 378–83,
    423–27
spiritual life, 269
stages of life, 78–80
strength, body, 141–51, 240–41
stress, 142, 148, 236–37, 242, 250–51,
    287–313, 418–19
stress incontinence. *See* leakage
stress, managing, 82, 100–101, 192, 244,
    252, 264, 268, 287–90, 292–313,
    316–17, 318–37, 342, 347, 385, 386,
    389–91, 398, 418–21
stroke, 74, 97–98, 103, 160, 161, 164, 222,
    267, 291, 298
success, 410–11
successful aging, 80

ABOUT THE AUTHOR

An award-winning journalist, bestselling author, motivational speaker, and women's health & wellness advocate, **Joan Lunden** has been a trusted voice in American homes for more than thirty years. For nearly two decades, Lunden greeted viewers each morning on *Good Morning America* bringing insight to the day's top stories. As the longest-running female host ever on early morning television, Lunden reported from twenty-six countries, covered five presidents, five Olympics, and kept Americans up to date on how to care for their homes, their families, and their health. As one of America's most recognized and trusted personalities, Lunden has graced the covers of more than seventy magazines and book covers. Through her website JoanLunden.com and her social media, she interacts with women across the country every day on topics from wellness, to survivorship, and aging. Joan's recent titles have included: special correspondent on the *TODAY* show, host of the CBS series *Your Health,* sought-after speaker and event host throughout the country, senior caregiving advocate, and, most recently, breast cancer survivor. Lunden documented her battle through cancer treatment and wrote a memoir *Had I Known* reflecting on her life and career. Lunden has served as national spokesperson for various organizations such as The American Heart Association, Mothers Against Drunk Driving, The American Lung Association, The American Red Cross, The American Academy of Pediatrics, and The Colon Cancer Alliance. Joan Lunden's books include *Had I Known; Chicken Soup for the Soul: Family Caregiving; Growing Up Healthy: Protecting Your Child from Diseases Now Through Adulthood; Wake-Up Calls; A Bend in the Road Is Not the End of the Road; Joan Lunden's Healthy Living; Joan Lunden's Healthy Cooking; Mother's Minutes; Your Newborn Baby;* and *Good Morning, I'm Joan Lunden.* She also hosts the exercise video *Workout America.*